Medical Complications
of
Quadriplegia

Medical Complications of Quadriplegia

PETER H. BERCZELLER, M.D., F.A.C.P.

Professor of Clinical Medicine
New York University School of Medicine
New York, New York

MARY F. BEZKOR, M.D.

Clinical Instructor of Physical Medicine and Rehabilitation
New York University School of Medicine
New York, New York

YEAR BOOK MEDICAL PUBLISHERS, INC.
Chicago • London

Library of Congress Cataloging-in-Publication Data

Berczeller, Peter H.
  Medical complications of quadriplegia.

  Includes bibliographies and index.
  1. Quadriplegia—Treatment. I. Bezkor, Mary. F.
II. Title. [DNLM: 1. Quadriplegia—complications.
WL 346 B486m]
RC406.Q33B47 1986   617'.58   85-26526
ISBN 0-8151-0700-5

Sponsoring Editor: Richard H. Lampert
Manager, Copyediting Services: Frances M. Perveiler
Production Project Manager: Carol Ennis Coghlan
Proofroom Supervisor: Shirley E. Taylor

1 2 3 4 5 6 7 8 9 0 K C 90, 89, 88, 87, 86

To the Memory of Samuel Repko, Jr.

Contributors

ANGELO R. CANEDO, PH.D.
Clinical Instructor of Psychiatry
New York University School of Medicine
New York, New York

PAUL R. COOPER, M.D.
Associate Professor of Neurosurgery
New York University School of Medicine
New York, New York

DAVID L. KAMELHAR, M.D.
Assistant Professor of Clinical Medicine
New York University School of Medicine
New York, New York

ZAFAR KHAN, M.D.
Assistant Professor of Urology
Mount Sinai School of Medicine
New York, New York

ARNOLD MELMAN, M.D.
Associate Professor of Urology
Mount Sinai School of Medicine
New York, New York

ROBERT A. PRESS, M.D., PH.D.
Instructor of Clinical Medicine
New York University School of Medicine
New York, New York

Foreword

Remarkable advances have occurred in the treatment of spinal cord injuries during the past 40 years. Based largely on experience gained in the fields of neurology, neurosurgery, and rehabilitation medicine, a considerable volume of data has accumulated. Both textbooks and the world medical literature have documented the transition from the early days—when fewer than 5% of men in the armed forces who incurred spinal cord injuries survived for more than a year after injury—to the present—when anticipated longevity of patients with spinal cord injuries is close to that of the general population.

Of the spectrum of spinal cord injuries, quadriplegia represents one of the most formidable challenges to even the most astute clinician. Rendering clinical services to quadriplegic patients requires the coordinated and cooperative efforts of a multidisciplinary medical group. The concept of organized team effort is the guiding principle of *Medical Management of Quadriplegia,* which is a thoughtful compilation of the viewpoints and approaches of physicians of various disciplines who are involved in the care of quadriplegic patients. The authors and contributors have created a pithy, important, information-filled work, which should serve to enhance and expand the resources of all colleagues, and especially those who encounter this catastrophic condition relatively infrequently in their specialties and practices.

JOSEPH GOODGOLD, M.D.
The Howard A. Rusk Professor and Chairman
Department of Rehabilitation Medicine
New York University School of Medicine
Director of Rehabilitation Medical Services
New York University Medical Center
New York, New York

Preface

The presentation of both common and uncommon problems of quadriplegia is distinctly out of the ordinary. In pediatrics there is a similar disparity between pathology and presentation. Whereas the pediatric patient is aware of pain but cannot communicate, the quadriplegic can communicate but cannot appreciate pain, distention of a viscus, heat, or any of the other sensations the ordinary patient experiences and upon which we depend so much in our evaluation of the clinical situation.

In a very real sense, the physician who cares for a quadriplegic must reorient his clinical thinking. He has to almost replace the history and instead emphasize the physical examination as well as the interpretation of the laboratory and other ancillary findings.

This book is designed to convey to all who take care of quadriplegics the crucial importance of meticulous, understanding, and sophisticated medical care.

One need not be a neurologist or neurosurgeon to have the necessary understanding of the distorted pathophysiology encountered in quadriplegics. We envisage that, with the increased survival of these patients, they will be cared for in much the same way as other patients, in their homes, doctors' offices, and community hospitals.

It is therefore that much more important that *all* physicians who care for general medical problems learn how to deal with the admittedly unusual but still ultimately predictable sequelae of spinal cord injury.

PETER H. BERCZELLER, M.D.
MARY F. BEZKOR, M.D.

Acknowledgments

Our thanks go to Joseph Goodgold, M.D., The Howard A. Rusk Professor and Chairman, Department of Rehabilitation Medicine, New York University School of Medicine, and Director of Rehabilitation Medical Services, New York University Medical Center, New York, New York, for his encouragement early in the course of this project. We also appreciate his painstaking and thorough review of the manuscript.

Our thanks go to Enid McNally for her faithful and thorough assistance with research and proofreading.

Mrs. Marian Saunders' clerical help is also very much appreciated.

PETER H. BERCZELLER, M.D.
MARY F. BEZKOR, M.D.

Contents

1

Initial Clinical Evaluation and Management

PAUL R. COOPER, M.D.

A HIGH DEGREE of suspicion is essential in order that injury to the cervical spine and spinal cord is not overlooked after trauma. As many as 10% of all patients with spinal injuries will develop new or progressive neurologic deficits during the initial stage of management—often from failure to recognize the presence or severity of bony injury.[10]

All patients who complain of neck pain after trauma—*no matter how trivial the injury appears*—should have a plain film examination. Similarly, patients who complain of weakness, hyperesthesias, dysesthesias, or paresthesias in the upper or lower extremities should be suspected of having a spinal cord injury. Patients whose level of consciousness is impaired as a result of head injury or shock must be suspected of having a cervical spine injury until proved otherwise.

A careful neurologic examination is essential to determine the presence of objective deficit and to serve as a baseline for evaluating subsequent improvement or deterioration.[8]

In the upper cervical spine (C1-C3) the spinal cord segments are opposite the same vertebral bodies. Below C4 the cervical spinal segment cord at any level is one-half to one level higher than the vertebral body of the same number.

Thus, the C7 spinal cord segment is opposite the C6 vertebral body. Nerve roots exit between adjacent vertebrae, and from C1–7 are numbered for the higher of the two vertebrae between which they exit. Thus, the C5 root exits between the C4 and C5 vertebrae. There are eight cervical nerve roots and cord segments and only seven cervical vertebrae; between the C7 and T1 bone segments, the nerve root that exits is the C8 root. Below this level the nerve root is numbered after the lower of the two vertebrae between which it exits.

Spinal cord injury at the T1 level will result in incomplete loss of function of the intrinsic hand muscles, including the interossei, lumbricals, and the abductor pollicis longus as well as all spinal cord innervated structures below this level. Injury at the C8 level will result in complete paralysis of the lumbricals and interossei muscles. At the C7 level the triceps muscle that controls extension of the forearms will be affected. Injuries at the C6 level will affect the biceps muscle that controls flexion of the forearm and is supplied by the C6 (and, to a lesser extent, the C5) nerve root. At the C5 level the deltoid muscle that controls abduction of the arms at the shoulders will be affected.

The diaphragm is supplied by spinal nerves C3–5. Thus, in patients who have spinal cord injuries at the C5 level and above, diaphragmatic movement will be compromised to varying degrees. Injury to the spinal cord above C3 will result in total respiratory muscle paralysis. In such patients, early intubation and mechanical ventilation are necessary to sustain life. Even in those patients with injury below C5, respiratory movement will be compromised because of paralysis of the intercostal muscles. Respiratory insufficiency may occur quite precipitously in patients with lesions below C5 as a result of fatiguing of the diaphragm, which must perform the entire work of respiration without the aid of the intercostal muscles. Frequent arterial blood gas studies will give the clinician early warning of a falling Po_2 and rising Pco_2 even when the patient is not in apparent respiratory distress.

Although there is some anatomic variation from patient to patient, the pattern of sensory loss is also helpful in delineating the level of injury. The undersurface of the proximal arm is supplied by T1; the fourth and fifth fingers and ulnar aspect of the palm are supplied by C8; the midpalm and middle finger by C7; the first two fingers, radial side of the palm, and forearm by C6; the shoulder by C5; the area just below the clavicle by C4; the lower neck by C3; and the upper neck to the angle of the mandible by C2.

In addition to motor and sensory changes, patients with complete lesions experience spinal shock with absence of deep tendon reflexes and muscular hypotonia. Spasticity gradually appears after three to four weeks with increased (nonvoluntary) muscle tone and hyperactive deep tendon reflexes.

Injury to sympathetic pathways in the ventrolateral white matter of the spinal cord commonly accompanies complete lesions. The clinical manifestations include hypotension to a moderate degree (70 to 90 mm Hg systolic) and bradycardia. Bradycardia is not seen in hypovolemic shock and serves to distinguish this entity from hypotension caused by trauma to sympathetic pathways in the spinal cord.

Ileus and fecal retention are also common in the acute phase. Urinary retention with a large hypotonic bladder is invariably seen with complete lesions and should be anticipated and treated early with catheterization of the bladder.

When there is incomplete motor or sensory loss, the remaining neurologic function sometimes fits into one of several syndromes. Schneider et al.[12] in 1954 described the central cervical spinal cord syndrome, which consists of relatively greater weakness in the arms as compared to the legs. Bladder involvement is inconsistent, and sensory changes are variable. The injury generally occurs following severe hyperextension in patients with narrow spinal canals and osteophytic ridges. The predominance of upper extremity motor deficit is due to the central location of these fibers in the cervical spinal cord. A varying degree of recovery is possible, but many patients are left with permanent deficit.

The syndrome of hemisection of the spinal cord was described by Brown-Sequard in 1850 and is manifest by motor deficit on the side of the lesion, ipsilateral loss of joint position sense, and contralateral loss of pain and temperature sensation beginning one or two segments below the level of the lesion.

At the level of trauma there will also be lower motor neuron deficits from injury to the anterior horn cells.

The syndrome of acute anterior spinal cord injury was described by Schneider in 1955.[11] It occurs as a result of spinal cord compression by herniated cervical discs or fracture-subluxations. Clinical features include total motor paralysis below the level of the lesion, decreased to absent pin sensation below the lesion, and the preservation of joint position sense.

Usually, none of these syndromes prevails and motor loss of varying degrees is present below the level of the injury accompanied by spotty sensory loss without apparent anatomic logic.

RADIOGRAPHIC EVALUATION

All patients who are suspected of having a cervical spine fracture or subluxation because of clinical signs or symptoms, should be treated as if a fracture or subluxation actually exists. Such patients should have their necks immobilized with a collar or have a piece of tape passed over their forehead to hold their heads firm to their bed or stretcher. If possible, the patient should not be moved and a portable x-ray should be taken in the lateral projection on the emergency room stretcher. The C7-T1 junction is often obscured by the shoulders in young husky males and can be visualized by pulling the patient's arms caudally or, if that is not helpful, by performing a swimmer's view.

The diagnostic evaluation of patients with spine injury has been summarized previously in an article by Maravilla et al.[9] In those patients whose films demonstrate fractures or subluxations but who do not have neurologic deficit, appropriate immobilization is established according to principles and techniques that are detailed in subsequent sections. In the past, full definition of the nature of the fracture has been obtained using polytomography. Recent experience with the CT scanner shows that this modality, when skillfully used, can identify fractures as accurately as polytomography. In general, myelography is not performed on patients without neurologic deficit.

In patients with neurologic deficit, the sequence and goals of the diagnostic evaluation are different. Immobilization is instituted in the same fashion as in those patients without deficit and plain films are obtained to define the level and nature of bony injury. In patients with complete loss of motor and sensory function below the level of the lesion, neurologic recovery of any significant degree is unlikely and further radiologic evaluation is limited to defining the pathologic anatomy of the fracture and/or subluxation at a convenient time using polytomograms or the CT scanner.

On the other hand, patients who have neurologic deficit with preservation of some motor or sensory function should have the earliest and most aggressive diagnostic evaluation to determine the presence of spinal cord compression. Plain films are first taken and the site of injury is defined. The patient is kept immobilized in the supine position, the subarachnoid space is punctured laterally at the C1–2 level, and 5 to 6 ml of metrizamide, a water-soluble contrast agent, is introduced. A myelogram is performed to determine the presence of spinal cord compression. If a high-resolution CT scanner is available, transaxial cuts are performed to further define the extent and nature (blood, disc, bone) of spinal cord compression and the anatomy of the bony injury.

The patient with incomplete neurologic deficit and apparently normal plain films presents a particularly difficult problem. The possible diagnoses are several. A small spinal canal with osteophytes that intrude on the canal may contuse the spinal cord in the absence of a fracture or subluxation, an intervertebral disc herniation may be present that cannot be seen on plain films, or a subluxation with spinal cord injury may have occurred at the time of trauma with reduction taking place prior to the time that cervical spine films are obtained. It is essential that all patients with incomplete neurologic deficit and normal cervical spine films have a metrizamide myelogram followed by CT scanning. If the myelogram is normal, plain x-rays in the lateral projection may be taken in extension and flexion to rule out the possibility of an occult subluxation.

BONY INJURY

The bony spine is most mobile in the cervical region. While this has the advantage of allowing a wide variety of movements of the head on the trunk, this mobility and lack of protection of the neck have the disadvantage of rendering the cervical spine vulnerable to injury. In normal circumstances the greatest movement of the cervical spine (and the entire spine for that matter) occurs between the C5–6 and C6–7 segments. It is thus understandable that these two segments are the commonest sites of fractures and subluxations.

The initial goal of management is immobilization of an unstable spine and reduction of fractures or subluxations. This generally can be achieved in the emergency room by the establishment of cervical traction. Until recently, Crutchfield tongs were the most common means of establishing traction. More recently, Crutchfield tongs have been superceded by Gardner-Wells tongs that have the advantage of being rapidly inserted without the necessity of incising the scalp or drilling holes in the skull. A third option for establishing cervical traction is the use of the halo ring, a round ribbon of stainless steel slightly larger in diameter than the head. It is secured to the head with four pins and has the advantage of being able to be connected to a plastic or plaster vest for long-term maintenance of stability.

Regardless of the type of apparatus used, a rope is connected to the device that fits over a pulley and is, in turn, connected to weights. The direction of traction is applied in the long axis of the body so as to keep the head in a neutral or slightly extended position. If necessary, more extension of the neck can be obtained by placing a folded sheet beneath the patient's shoulder or by inserting the tongs more anteriorly in the patient's head. Flexion, on the other hand, has the effect of increasing most subluxations and narrowing the upper cervical spinal canal at the site of the fracture, and should be avoided.

Patients in cervical traction may be turned from side to side for bathing, changing of bedding, or to prevent skin breakdown. These positional changes should not affect alignment of fractures as long as the relative flexion or extension of the cervical spine is not altered. Similarly, the head of the patient's bed may be raised or lowered as long as the direction of traction is maintained to prevent flexion or extension of the patient's neck.

FACET DISLOCATION

Bilateral facet dislocation results from a severe flexion injury. There is disruption of the facet joint complex and the intervertebral disc space. Neurologic deficit is generally profound. With bilateral facet dislocations, subluxations are generally severe. Unilateral facet dislocation occurs from a combination of rotatory and flexion forces and is often associated with no neurologic deficit. Lateral x-rays will show the superior facet of the lower vertebra to be lying posterior to the inferior facet of the upper vertebra. Treatment consists of insertion of cervical tongs or halo traction with gradually increasing weight to effect reduction. Often reduction is achieved only after traction with 60 to 80 lb of weight.

Even if reduction is achieved, these subluxations remain unstable and reduction will often be lost if halo-vest immobilization is attempted. Moreover, even if stability is maintained, ligamentous healing frequently fails to occur after two or three months. For this reason, patients with such injuries are treated with posterior cervical wiring and fusion with iliac crest bone grafts. In the postoperative period, patients are placed in a collar for three months until fusion takes place.

VERTEBRAL BODY FRACTURES

Mild compression fractures of the vertebral bodies occur from axial loading. These fractures are generally stable and, if not associated with neurologic deficit, may be treated with immobilization with a Philadelphia collar.

With more severe axial loading (particularly in the presence of slight flexion) a burst fracture of the vertebral body is produced with retropulsion of the body and disc into the spinal canal with compression of the spinal cord. The exact anatomy of the injury can be defined by metrizamide myelography followed by high-resolution CT scanning. Treatment consists of anterior decompression with excision of the shattered vertebral body and disc fragments with decompression of the spinal cord.[3] An iliac crest bone graft is placed at the site of the vertebrectomy. Postoperative immobilization is maintained using a halo-vest apparatus.

In patients with burst fractures without spinal cord compression, immobilization in a halo-vest may result in healing and stability. These patients must be followed carefully after the removal of the halo immobilization, since progressive kyphotic deformity sometimes occurs. For this reason some authors choose to treat these injuries with vertebrectomy and iliac crest bone grafting even if neural compression is not present.[4]

CONCLUSION

Few diseases or injuries have the potential for producing the devastating effects on survival and quality of life that cervical spinal cord trauma does. Despite the vast amount of research, there is currently no medical treatment that has been proven effective in ameliorating the effects of mechanical injury to the spinal cord.

Current management consists of early recognition of the injury, immobilization of the spine, reduction of subluxations, and prevention of further injury. Diagnostic evaluation has two goals: the definition of the pathologic anatomy of the fracture or subluxation, and the determination of the presence of spinal cord compression.

Patients with spinal cord compression and incomplete neurologic deficit should have decompression and spinal stabilization. Patients with neurologic deficit who do not have spinal cord compression are stabilized using operative or nonoperative means, as appropriate. Patients with total sensorimotor loss below the level of their lesion rarely, if ever, recover significant function even if decompression is achieved. Operative stabilization is performed in these patients to minimize bony deformities and prevent the progression of neurological deficit.

REFERENCES

1. Alexander E., Davis C.H.: Reduction and fusion of fracture of the odontoid process. *J. Neurosurg.* 31:580, 1969.
2. Apuzzo M.L.J., Heiden J.S., Weiss M.H., et al.: Acute fractures of the odontoid process: An analysis of 45 cases. *J. Neurosurg.* 48:85, 1978.
3. Bohlmann H.H., Eismont F.J.: Surgical techniques of anterior decompression and fusion for spinal cord injuries. *Clin. Orthop.* 154:57, 1981.
4. Bohlmann H.H., Freehofer A.A., DeJaks J.J.: Late anterior decompression of spinal cord injuries: A report of 36 cases. *J. Bone Joint Surg.* 57A:1025, 1975.
5. Cooper P.R., Maravilla K.R., Sklar F.H., et al.: Halo immobilization of cervical spine fractures: Indications and results. *J. Neurosurg.* 50:603, 1979.
6. Effendi B., Roy D., Cornish B., et al.: Fracture of the ring of the atlas: A classification based on the analysis of 131 cases. *J. Bone Joint Surg.* 63B:319, 1981.
7. Jefferson G.: Fracture of the atlas vertebra: Report of 4 cases and a review of those previously recorded. *Br. J. Surg.* 7:407, 1920.
8. McQueen J.D., Khan M.I.: Evaluation of patients with cervical spine lesions, in Cervical Spine Research Society: *The Cervical Spine.* Philadelphia, J.B. Lippincott Co., 1983, pp. 128–146.
9. Maravilla K.R., Cooper P.R., Sklar F.H.: The influence of thin-section tomography on the treatment of cervical spine injuries. *Radiology* 127:131, 1978.
10. Rogers W.A.: Fractures and dislocations of the cervical spine: An end result study. *J. Bone Joint Surg.* 39A:34, 1957.
11. Schneider R.C.: The syndrome of acute anterior spinal cord injury. *J. Neurosurg.* 12:95, 1955.
12. Schneider R.C., Cherry G., Pantek H.: The syndrome of acute central cervical spinal cord injury with special reference to the mechanism involved in hyperextension injuries of the cervical spine. *J. Neurosurg.* 11:546, 1954.
13. Seljeskog E.L., Chou S.N.: Spectrum of the hangman's fracture. *J. Neurosurg.* 45:3, 1976.

2

The Psychological Impact of Spinal Cord Injury

ANGELO R. CANEDO, Ph.D.

A SPINAL CORD INJURY is clearly a major trauma, and treatment requires specific care strategies. The medical implications of such an injury are extensive. While the emotional impact of such trauma is not discounted, it is evident that the first focus of attention for both the patient and the medical staff should be on the physical sequelae of the injury.

As the aspects of acute medical care retreat into the background, the emotional reactions often become more pronounced and begin to assume more obvious importance to all parties concerned. Psychological reactions, frequently described as stages of adjustment, at times seem to parallel the process of medical care and can support the primary objective of preserving life.

These emotional reactions can often serve to maximize the potential for recovery. On the other hand, some of the specific emotional reactions that patients with spinal cord injury experience may conflict with or even hamper medical efforts at rehabilitation. Therefore, as the recovery process unfolds, the individual's psychological adjustment may pose a major barrier that needs to be overcome before the patient can return to some form of productive life.[11, 20, 38, 48]

EPIDEMIOLOGY

Spinal cord injuries are rather infrequent disabilities compared with other major medical conditions, yet they are seriously debilitating and extremely costly. The available data on spinal cord injuries are drawn mostly from surveys conducted during the 1970s.[7,47] One of these major surveys was based on data obtained from a nationwide compilation of hospital discharge reports. The estimates of incidence are about five new spinal cord injury cases per 100,000 of population per year. Direct and indirect care costs for these individuals were estimated to be about $234 million in 1974 and extrapolated to be about $380 million in 1980 dollars. The average cost per year when averaging acute and ongoing care patients was $8,800 per person in 1974, or about $14,390 per person in 1980 dollars.

INCIDENCE OF SPINAL CORD INJURIES

The incidence of spinal cord injuries appears to be rising.[7] The incidence in 1970 was 29.1 per million inhabitants of the United States, while in 1977 it rose to 42.8 per million. Given the demographic breakdown of incidence and the most common causes of injury, one can postulate that an increasing number of older persons, along with the increasing use of motor vehicles by adolescents and young adults, are major factors influencing the rise in incidence.

GROUPS AT RISK

Males between the ages of 20 and 34 are at highest risk for spinal cord injury.[7] The incidence is as high as 68.0 per million among 20- to 24-year-olds, then drops gradually to a rate of 41.4 per million in 50- to 64-year-olds. The incidence then climbs again to a rate of 54.9 per million in the 65-plus age group. There are also some data (obtained in the late 1970s) that indicate a tremendous rise in the incidence of spinal cord injury among 15- to 19-year-old males, with speculation that this group at the time had the highest incidence of spinal cord injury.[47]

SEX AND RACE DATA

The ratio of males to females in the survey populations was 2.4 to 1. In the survey of hospital discharges, 69.2% were males while 30.8% were females. A survey sample breakdown by race indicated that 77.7% were white. The other racial groups only comprised 22.3% of the population. However, both surveys[7, 47] indicated a more recent rise in the rate of incidence among black males and noted that they are at twice the risk of white males.[7] Sports injuries are the most common cause of spinal cord injuries among white males, while penetrating wounds account for the greatest source of injuries among black males.[47]

COMMON CAUSES OF SPINAL CORD INJURIES

Motor vehicle injuries are the most common overall cause of spinal cord injuries. Forty-seven percent of the injuries reported were related to a motor vehicle accident.[47] These accidents were reported to be the most common cause for spinal cord injury resulting in paraplegia and quadriplegia.

Twenty-one percent of injuries were related to falls, and a large part of this group was elderly. Fifteen percent were sports related, and 13% were due to penetrating wounds. Sports injuries more commonly resulted in quadriplegia, while penetrating wounds often led to paraplegia.

FATALITY RATE

The hospital fatality rate for spinal cord injuries was 11.2%. Fatality was 36% more common in males and increased with age to a rate of 35.9% for men older than 65.[7]

Correlating Physical and Emotional Recovery

Poor neurologic recovery of function at the time of hospital discharge seems to be correlated with poor emotional adjustment or adaptation to the physical trauma.[6] Research indicates that persons who experienced severe sensory loss at the time of discharge were less positive about the future than were persons with less residual sensory deficit. Patients with severe motor loss at the time of discharge had less so-called ego resilience or internal strength when compared with those patients experiencing less motor loss upon discharge.

INITIAL ADJUSTMENT: THE SHOCK REACTION

The reaction of emotional shock frequently has been described as the initial response to spinal cord injury.[4] This response is usually concurrent with the period of critical care during the first few days or weeks after a spinal cord injury. There are many opinions covering a wide range of possibilities as to what might account for this observed shock reaction.

Neurophysiologic Factors

Some clinicians have speculated that there are major biochemical and physiologic changes present following spinal cord injury.[21] Others question whether the changes noted in some of these patients may be due to a closed head injury that occurred simultaneously with the spinal cord injury.[34] In addition, with upper cord injuries there are often potential effects on cognition and mentation due to respiratory involvement.[1] Yet another factor that may play a major role in the etiology of the patient's change in mentation is the presence of side effects of the medications being given to these individuals for pain, spasticity, and so on.[1]

ENVIRONMENTAL FACTORS

Behavioral researchers believe that the sensory deprivation the individual experiences shortly after a major injury often leads to some of the observed confusion or mental clouding.[44] They cite the literature on syndromes such as ICU psychosis and stimulus deprivation as support.

EMOTIONAL FACTORS

The initial confrontation with spinal cord injury is an emotionally harrowing experience. Some authors describe the spinal-cord-injured patient as experiencing emotional defenses such as denial in its most extreme form and note that the emotional shock serves as a much-needed defense. This first reaction represents an acute emotional crisis,[40] with shock being a normal emotional defense that can allow the individual time for emotional regrouping.

THEORIES OF PSYCHOLOGICAL ADJUSTMENT

Many of the initial theories on adjustment to a spinal cord injury used frameworks directly adopted from previously existing theories of personality and emotional adjustment. These theories, which were initially developed to help explain emotional reactions to issues such as separation, loss, and death, were often unable to address the specific reactions to severe physical disability. While many clinicians adhere to different aspects or approaches derived from these theories, a series of theoretical formulations has developed that attempts to more accurately describe the process of adjustment to a physical disability.

A major drawback to this work is that most of the theories have not been empirically based and are actually based on clinical impressions.

Emotional adjustment theories have three major foci.[37] The first group of theories has an intrapsychic focus and addresses the process of adjustment by concentrating on the reactions of the disabled person to the world around him. The second group of theories focuses on how the individual copes with the personal loss and how he can work with the world around him. The third group takes a social change model, arguing for fair opportunity and social acceptance as the key factors in adjustment.

INTRAPERSONAL MODELS

The Kübler-Ross Model

The theory most commonly referred to when clinicians speak of adjusting to a disability is that proposed by Elisabeth Kübler-Ross in describing the process of the acceptance of one's own death or that of a significant other.[32] Although not solidly founded in empirical research, her theory is based on the clinical summaries and impressions of more than 200 patients and their families. She describes a process that begins with denial and isolation, a "No! Not me!" reaction. Here the individual often does not accept or believe the practical information or prognosis being extended to him by medical personnel. These patients either selectively hear the information being given to them or simply choose to deny the opinions offered.

The second stage of adjustment is marked by feelings of intense anger and resentment depicted in comments such as "Why me?" During this stage, nursing personnel often find the patient difficult to work with on a daily basis. The individual is often described by staff as being cynical, negative, abrasive, intolerant, and demanding.

The third stage is one of bargaining in an attempt to postpone or get rid of the overwhelming problem. This third stage is frequently a difficult one for medical personnel because the patient will often question medical procedure or even doubt the physician's clinical judgment and prognosis. According to Kübler-Ross, when coping with death, much of the bargaining occurs with God. In contrast, the spinal-cord-injured person who has a reasonably full life ahead of him but is faced with motor and/or sensory deficits does a large part of his bargaining with medical science as well.

The fourth stage is that of depression. This stage is characterized by many of the reactions common to emotional withdrawal and social isolation. These reactions so commonly ascribed to depression will be detailed in a later section.

The fifth and final stage is that of acceptance. Here the individual begins to take a fresh look at his physical limitations. With this new perspective he can try to get on with his life.

While there are no specific time frames set for these adjustment stages, most clinicians would say that they usually take from six months to three years before a patient completes them successfully. The time frames for each of the substages are variable and depend on the individual.

Some Additional Intrapersonal Views

Many other theorists and researchers have highlighted adjustment issues.* Each addresses a particular stage or reaction and more specifically details an individual's response. A review of these articles is outside the purview of this chapter, and the reader is referred to the reference list for more extensive reading.

There is one slightly different perspective that will be noted here since it has gained increased attention in the recent literature. The opinion varies slightly but seems to be that many disabled persons will often react in the same way to a disability but then bounce back to their premorbid selves after about six months. The reactions during this adjustment period are often described as extreme but reasonably appropriate and predictable given the severity of the loss.[33] As a point of departure, the work of Kübler-Ross indicates that the individual first experiences denial. This reaction is commonly thought to last anywhere from three to eight weeks, although it may take longer. The denial is then followed closely by a significant

*See references, 4, 6, 25, 30, 33, 35, 41, 43, 49, 50.

depression that is frequently characterized by withdrawal. Time frames for this stage vary widely. The bargaining that ensues in the next stage is often accompanied by a seemingly aggressive or confrontational style that is thought by many to be part of an agitated depression. Subsequently, there is a gradual return to normal.[28]

The most common emotions that have been observed in recently disabled persons are anxiety and depression.[41] These often take the form of uncontrollable affect, egocentricity, and a potential explosiveness.[4] These reactions seem to be based on personal unrest and irritability secondary to a sense of personal powerlessness.

Some authors have described initial autistic-like reactions that resemble behavioral and emotional freeze states.[4] These are coupled with unrealistic thinking about life problems and with seemingly impaired judgement over a period of time. Others report that aggression and rebellion are the reactions following grief, fear, and anxiety.[31] In addition, some have described a passivity, dependence, and submissiveness that alternates with and sharply contrasts with the demanding behavior previously described. As the process resolves, these patients become increasingly ambivalent and ultimately begin to reassume personal responsibility.

Behavioral Models

During the period of severe depression described by Kübler-Ross, the individual often experiences a number of personal reactions. These are common enough reactions, but they may require modification through professional assistance and monitoring to assure that they do not go beyond the common limits of expression. The reactions common to depression are shown in Table 2–1. While these are common reactions, as previously noted, they are evaluated for their appropriateness in terms of degree. When in doubt as to the appropriateness of an individual's response, it is often a good idea to consult a mental health colleague such as a rehabilitation psychologist or consulting psychiatrist.

TABLE 2–1.—REACTIONS COMMON
TO DEPRESSION*

Sadness
Pessimism
Sense of failure
Dissatisfaction
Guilt
Expectation of punishment
Self-dislike
Self-accusation
Ideas or fantasies of self-harm
Isolation fantasies and fears
Crying
Irritability
Social withdrawal
Indecisiveness
Changes in body image
Vegetative signs
   Changes in eating and sleeping behavior
   Changes in general fatigue level
Somatic preoccupation
Issues/concerns pertaining to sexuality

*Adapted from Beck A.: *Depression: Causes and Treatment.* Philadelphia, University of Pennsylvania Press, 1967.

VARYING EMOTIONAL REACTIONS OF THE SPINAL CORD INJURED

Not all patients demonstrate the previously detailed reactions after a spinal cord injury, and the absence of the many strong emotional reactions listed in the table is not considered particularly out of the norm by some authors.[15] Several studies have compared disabled patients with a group of same aged able-bodied peers and found no differences in their emotional profiles as measured by common personality tests.[10, 46]

Although depression may be an extremely common reaction, its absence does not always imply denial of the disability and is therefore not an indicator of maladjustment. It appears that those persons with spinal cord injury who do not seem to experience a significant depression are often those who cope best with the overall impact of the disability.[47]

Issues in Social Adjustment

Recently, some emphasis has been placed on the emotional impact of facing the problems of social inequality. This has been joined with efforts to achieve architectural accessibility and to remove other environmental barriers to equal access. The thrust has been in the direction of the achievement of change in social attitudes. Some authors have said that the realization of these personal and social barriers is at times the primary reason for the many severe emotional reactions observed after a newfound disability.[24] Thus, from a more social perspective, depression results from the loss of access to opportunities for reinforcement.[18, 39]

The result of the many social pressures that arise is the existence of a disabled community that is sheltered and isolated from the realities of life. These pressures often engender genuine emotional reactions of frustration, depression, and a sense of futility. From a psychosocial viewpoint these emotional responses are not pathological. It is felt that these are appropriate reactions to what is often perceived as a hopeless situation.

CONCLUSION

While there are many components and specific emotional reactions to physical disability, most theorists agree on a series of specific stages. Each theorist labels these stages differently, depending on the emotional component of the reaction he or she wishes to highlight. However, the major stages remain much like those originally postulated.

Most authors agree that patients with spinal cord injury go through an initial shock reaction. There is a rather intense psychological disequilibrium that frequently accompanies other neurophysiologic and biochemical changes. These changes may at times lead to altered mentation.

The next stage is commonly defined as denial and is often characterized by an emotional retreat from the startling reality and impact of the disability. The individual is usually shaken by the implications of the disability on his life-style. Some authors believe that there is a total denial of the reality. Others think that there may be some awareness present but that these patients react to their symptoms as if they were only temporary. Most agree that as this defense system breaks down, the individual begins to exhibit anxiety, anger, and obvious common signs of depression. This breakdown of denial is deemed to be the first step in entering a period of acknowledgment.

Acknowledgment can last for a period of months or even years. The patient is now described as beginning to confront the realities of his disability. The obstacles faced and the problems addressed are individually selected and tend to be confronted at a pace and at a level with which the patient is comfortable. The process becomes one of working within the limitations imposed by the disability.

The final stage is that of adjustment. This stage is often not reached until several years after the onset of the disability, if it is reached at all. At this point, the individual has begun to effectively integrate the disability into his overall way of life. In many cases, these persons have had to make major adjustments in their lives and have developed new areas of interest and activity. Effective adjustment is achieved when the individual successfully incorporates the disability in proportion to the other aspects of his personality.

REFERENCES

1. Adams R., Victor M.: *Principles of Neurology.* New York, Mc-Graw-Hill Book Co., 1981.
2. Barber J., Adrian C.: *Psychological Approaches to the Management of Pain.* New York, Brunner/Mazel, 1982.
3. Beck A.: *Depression: Causes and Treatment.* Philadelphia, University of Pennsylvania Press, 1967.
4. Berger S., Garrett J.: Psychological problems of the paraplegic patient. *J. Rehabil.* 18:15–17, 1952.
5. Bracken M., Freedman D., Hellenbrand K.: Incidence of acute traumatic hospitalized spinal cord injuries in the United States, 1970–1977. *Am. J. Epidemiol.* 113:615–622, 1978.
6. Bracken M., Shepard M.: Coping and adaptation following acute spinal cord injury: A theoretical analysis. *Paraplegia* 18:74–85, 1980.
7. Bracken M., Shepard M., Webb S.: Psychological response to

acute spinal cord injury: An epidemiological study. *Paraplegia* 19:271–283, 1981.

8. Callaway E., Dembo D.: Narrowed attention. *Arch. Neurol. Psychiatry* 79:74–90, 1958.

9. Calliet R.: Chronic pain: Is it necessary? *Arch. Phys. Med. Rehabil.* 60:4–7, 1979.

10. Conomy J.: Disorders of body image after spinal cord injury. *Neurology* 23:842–850, 1973.

11. Cook D.: Psychological adjustment to spinal cord injury: Incidence of denial, depression and anxiety. *Rehabil. Psychol.* 26:97–104, 1979.

12. Cowen E.: Stress reduction and problem-solving rigidity. *J. Consult. Psychol.* 16:425–428, 1952.

13. Cull J., Hardy R.: *Behavior Modification in Rehabilitation Settings.* Springfield, Ill., Charles C Thomas Publisher, 1974.

14. Diethelm O., Jones M.: Influence of anxiety on attention, learning, retention and thinking. *Arch. Neurol. Psychiatry* 58:325–336, 1947.

15. Dinardo Q.: *Psychological Adjustment to Spinal Cord Injury,* dissertation. University of Houston, 1971.

16. Fair P., Basmajian J.: *Relaxation Therapy in Physical Medicine.* New York, Biomonitoring Applications Inc., 1976.

17. Fink S.: Crisis and motivation: A theoretical model. *Arch. Phys. Med. Rehabil.,* November 1966, pp. 592–597.

18. Fordyce W.: Behavioral methods in rehabilitation, in Neff W. (ed.): *Rehabilitation Psychology.* Washington, D.C., American Psychological Association, 1971.

19. Fordyce W.: *Behavioral Methods for Chronic Pain and Illness.* St. Louis, C.V. Mosby Co., 1976.

20. Garrett J., Levine E.: *Rehabilitation Practices with the Physically Disabled.* New York, Columbia University Press, 1973.

21. Grynbaum B.: Bellevue Hospital Medical Rounds, personal communication, spring 1983.

22. Grzesiak R.: Relaxation techniques in treatment of chronic pain. *Arch. Phys. Med. Rehabil.* 58:270–272, 1977.

23. Grzesiak R.: Rehabilitation of chronic pain syndromes, in Golden C. (ed.): *Current Topics in Rehabilitation Psychology.* New York, Grune & Stratton, 1984.

24. Hahn H.: Understanding psychosocial adjustment to disability through scientific research and the laboratory within. *Rehabil. Brief,* 7:1–4, 1984.

25. Hamburg D., Hamburg B., DeGoza S.: Adaptive problems and

mechanisms in severely burned patients. *Psychiatry* 16:1–20, 1953.

26. Hansell N.: *The Person in Distress.* New York, Human Sciences Press, 1976.

27. Hardy A., Elson R., Osmond-Clarke H.: *Practical Management of Spinal Cord Injuries.* New York, Churchill-Livingston, 1976.

28. Hohmann G.: Psychological aspects of rehabilitation of the spinal injured person. *Clin. Orthop.* 112:81–88, 1975.

29. Kalsbuk W., McLaurin R., Harris B., et al.: The national head and spinal cord injury survey: Major findings. *J. Neurosurg.* 53:S19-S31, 1980.

30. Kerr N.: Understanding the process of adjustment to disability, in Stubbins J. (ed.): *Social and Psychological Aspects of Disability.* Baltimore, Md., University Park Press, 1977.

31. Kerr W., Thompson M.: Acceptance of disability of sudden onset in paraplegia. *Int. J. Paraplegia.* 10:94–102, 1972.

32. Kübler-Ross E.: *On Death and Dying.* New York, Macmillan Publishing Co., 1969.

33. Mueller A.: Psychological factors in rehabilitation of paraplegic patients. *Arch. Phys. Med. Rehabil.* 43:151–159, 1962.

34. Murali L., Sokolow J., Grynbaum B.: Bellevue Hospital Medical Rounds. Personal communication, spring 1981.

35. Nagler B.: Psychiatric aspects of cord injury. *Am. J. Psychiatry* 107:49–56, 1951.

36. Richards J., Meredith R., Nepomuceno C., et al.: Psychosocial aspects of chronic pain in spinal cord injury. *Pain* 8:151–162, 1980.

37. Russell R.: Concepts of adjustment to disability: An overview. *Rehabil. Lit.* 42:330–337, 1981.

38. Rusk H.: *A World To Care For.* New York, Random House, 1977.

39. Seligman M.: *Helplessness: On Depression, Development and Death.* San Francisco, W.H. Freeman & Co., 1975.

40. Shumsky D.: Psychological and cognitive reactions in acute spinal cord injury, a doctoral dissertation proposal submitted to Bellevue Hospital and Rutgers University, fall 1984.

41. Siller J.: Psychological situation of the disabled with spinal cord injuries. *Rehabil. Lit.* 30:290–296, 1969.

42. Sternback R.: Pain and depression, in Kiev A. (ed.): *Somatic Manifestations of Depressive Disorders.* Princeton, N.J., Excerpta Medica, 1974, pp. 107–119.

43. Stone G., Cohen F., Adler N.: *Health Psychology—A Handbook.* Washington, D.C., Jossey-Bass, 1980.

44. Symington D., Fordyce W.: Changing concepts in the management of traumatic paraplegia. *Gen. Pract.* 32:141–155, 1965.
45. Taplin J.: Crisis theory: Critique and reformulation. *Community Ment. Health J.* 7:13–23, 1971.
46. Taylor G.: Predicted vs. actual response to spinal cord injury: A psychological study, dissertation. University of Minnesota, 1967.
47. Trieschmann R.: *Spinal Cord Injuries: Psychological, Social and Vocational Adjustment.* New York, Pergammon Press, 1982.
48. Trieschmann R.: The psychological aspects of spinal cord injury, in Golden C. (ed.): *Current Topics in Rehabilitation Psychology.* New York, Grune & Stratton, 1984.
49. Tucker S.: The psychology of spinal cord injury: Patient-staff interaction. *Rehabil. Lit.* 41:114–121, 1980.
50. Weller D., Miller P.: Emotional reactions of patient family and staff in the acute care period of spinal cord injury, pt. I. *Social Work in Health Care* 2:369–377, 1977.
51. Wittkower E., Gringas G., Mergler L., et al.: A combined psychosocial study of spinal cord lesions. *Can. Med. Assoc. J.* 71:109–115, 1954.

3

Respiratory Care

DAVID L. KAMELHAR, M.D.

CARDIOPULMONARY PROBLEMS rank high among the causes of death in quadriplegics both during the acute phase and also in later years.[17] The physician should assume that all quadriplegics have some degree of respiratory compromise.[24] For this reason, all internists caring for quadriplegic patients must be familiar with proper respiratory care both in theory and in practice.[8, 23]

The following chapter will outline pathophysiologic and clinical aspects of the team approach to acute and long-term care of the quadriplegic patient. Acute problems arising in the chronic quadriplegic patient will of course mandate measures outlined in those sections focusing on problems seen immediately following spinal cord injury.

PHYSIOLOGY

The muscles of respiration are of three groups: the diaphragm, intercostal and accessory muscles, and the abdominal muscles. Each muscle group has both inspiratory and expiratory function.[24]

Diaphragmatic contraction by downward displacement of abdominal viscera and outward displacement of the abdominal wall results in increased abdominal pressure. Simultaneous upward and outward displacement of the rib cage results from both direct diaphragmatic articulation with the rib cage and the increased abdominal pressure. Resulting negative pleural pressure thus leads to passive lung inflation. Under physiologic circumstances, the diaphragm is thus predominantly an inspiratory muscle and is the major muscle of respiration during quiet breathing. Diaphragmatic innervation is from phrenic nerves that arise from C-4. C-3 and C-5 provide accessory innervation.

Internal and external intercostal muscle fibers are innervated from the thoracic spine. Accessory muscles include scalenes, sternocleidomastoids, and trapezius. These are all inspiratory muscles. Although the upper external intercostals may be active during quiet respiration, the lower intercostals and accessories normally become active only at higher levels of ventilation.

Abdominal muscles of respiration are predominantly expiratory in function and facilitate passive lung recoil, especially during deep and forceful breathing. In the upright posture, abdominal muscle contraction lengthens the diaphragm, resulting in increased intra-abdominal pressure. Inspiration is thus assisted.[24]

In cervical quadriplegia, lower intercostal and abdominal muscles lose function. Accessory and intercostal muscles remain active. It has been observed in quadriplegics that up to 90% of total ventilation is contributed by accessory muscle contraction.[26] Diaphragmatic function is usually preserved; the extent of damage to C-3 and C-5 will determine the degree to which such function will be present.

Abdominal muscular flaccidity interferes with the contracting diaphragm's ability to create a positive intra-abdominal pressure. Failure of the paralyzed respiratory muscles to stabilize the chest wall against diaphragmatic contraction results in paradoxical advantage toward the supine position over the usually preferred erect position. In the erect or sitting position, the flaccid abdominal muscles allow the abdominal contents to fall. Thus, the diaphragm will be in a disadvantaged position for optimal contraction. In the supine position, abdominal contents elevate the diaphragm into the chest and thus optimize its fiber length for contraction. Therefore, abdominal binding to buttress the abdominal wall is useful for such patients when they must assume the erect position.[24, 26]

LUNG VOLUMES

Respiratory sequelae of neuromuscular disease are a result of the continued inspiratory and expiratory impairments described above. In cervical quadriplegia, the total lung capacity (TLC) is initially only modestly decreased. Normal recoil relationships of lung to chest wall maintain the lung's resting end expiratory volume or functional residual capacity (FRC) at midpoint. Residual volume (RV) approximates FRC; that is, the amount of air in the lung that can never be exhaled is approximately 50% of total lung capacity. Paralysis of expiratory muscles results in markedly diminished expiratory reserve volume (ERV) and cough capability. Inspiratory capacity (IC) is initially modestly diminished to 60% to 70% of baseline, with some return several months after injury.[3, 26] This improvement is the result of stabilization of the upper thoracic cage by spasticity of the involved respiratory muscles.[2, 27] Values of both vital capacity and maximal inspiratory pressure improve significantly in nine to ten weeks after injury, but no improvement in expiratory pressure is noted.[27]

Maximal inspiratory and expiratory pressures may be taken as indices of inspiratory and expiratory muscle strength, respectively. Values are depressed significantly at time of injury with 50% to 75% improvement in inspiratory pressure and 25% improvement in expiratory pressure determinations at 18 weeks.[27] Inspiratory pressures of less than -20 cm H_2O are classically taken as insufficient to maintain spontaneous ventilation in the otherwise intact patient and in the nonquadriplegic patient with acute respiratory failure.

GAS EXCHANGE

Varying degrees of gas exchange abnormality may be seen in quadriplegia, although relative preservation of normal pH,

Po_2, and Pco_2 is present in stable quadriplegics.[26, 27] Diffusing capacity is usually normal as well. The results of regional ventilation studies suggest a ventilation perfusion (V/Q) imbalance similar to that seen in small airways disease. Ineffective cough and chronic airway infection are likely mechanisms. Acute or severe infection as well as chronic underlying parenchymal or airways disease will further impair gas exchange by this mechanism. Various degrees of hypoxemia and hypercarbia will result.[2]

The central respiratory centers appear to respond nearly normally to peripheral stimuli of hypoxemia and hypercarbia in stable quadriplegics.[26] Chronic derangements in gas exchange on the basis of combined neuromuscular and airway dysfunction may blunt normal central responses to hypoxemia and hypercarbia, as is seen in other states of chronic alveolar hypoventilation.[3]

Mechanics and Work of Breathing

The marked increase in work of breathing makes fatigue and respiratory failure of great concern in the care of the quadriplegic.[3, 16]

Work of breathing is increased since nearly all muscles of respiration are nonfunctional except for the diaphragm. Abdominal wall flaccidity necessitates greater than normal transdiaphragmatic effort to achieve positive intra-abdominal pressure. Paradoxical rib cage motion during inspiration compounds the problem, particularly during the early months of quadriplegia. Post-traumatic intercostal muscle spasticity often alleviates this added factor.[27]

Coupled with these changes in chest wall mechanics are alterations in lung compliance that result from inability to expand the lung fully. The observation that maximum breathing capacity (MBC), peak flow, and maximal midexpiratory flow rates are depressed by only 40% is explained by a coupling of absent expiratory muscles with normal airway conductance. Ventilation at the highest achievable lung volume will thus permit elastic recoil properties of lung and chest wall to passively conduct the expiratory phase of ventilation. It is further apparent that impairment of airway conductance, as would be seen in obstructive airways disease, would significantly disrupt this favorable relationship. Sigh or periodic hyperinflation usually reappears in the subacute phase of quadriplegia. There is better clearing of airway secretions in the presence of these periodic hyperinflations and hence fewer serious respiratory infections.[26]

ALTERATIONS IN SENSATION OF DYSPNEA IN QUADRIPLEGICS

It has been observed that patients with high spinal cord transection (C2) may lack the sensation of dyspnea in response to apnea as might occur with ventilator malfunction.[34] Backup alarm for such failure should be utilized.

Patients who experience generalized spasm as may occur following positioning may experience simultaneous dyspnea.[37] The dyspnea lasts for the duration of the spasm and is caused by diaphragmatic spasm with the diaphragm maintained in inspiration. Expiration begins with the end of the spasm and diaphragmatic relaxation.

COUGH

Adequate pulmonary toilet and clearing of secretions depend on a complex interaction of the respiratory musculature. The initial phase of cough normally includes a deep inspiration that is followed by a compressive phase. Following glottic closure, the expiratory phase begins with glottic opening and requires further contraction of expiratory muscles to maintain high pressure and flow rates with expulsion of respiratory secretions. A series of consecutive coughs at progressively smaller lung volumes moves secretions from small to larger airways. A second deep breath and cough will then expel these more centralized secretions.[21]

Inability to perform this series of maneuvers successfully because of both inspiratory and expiratory muscle weakness will (logically) result in retained secretions. Ventilation perfusion mismatches described above will result in chronic low-grade gas exchange abnormality. Acute or chronic increases in secretions and combined mechanisms for depressed cough may result in recurrent infection, ventilatory failure, or both, necessitating assisted ventilation.[17, 27, 33]

ACUTE CARE

EARLY EVALUATION

Respiratory evaluation and care of the acute spinal-cord-injured patient must begin at the time and place of injury. On-the-scene recognition of present or impending respiratory failure supercedes the urgency of speedy evacuation to a medical facility.[17, 28]

Upon arrival at the emergency room, respiratory pattern and neurologic and mental statuses should be evaluated along with monitoring of basic vital signs.

An impaired level of consciousness, in addition to traumatic brain injury, should suggest the presence of a toxic suppressive substance in the patient's blood that may have caused the accident. Respiratory compromise on a central basis may result.

Trauma to the nose or mouth may result in obstruction of the upper airway, either directly or by aspiration of blood, teeth, tongue, or nonfixed prosthodontic devices. The presence of vomitus should suggest aspiration of gastric contents into the tracheobronchial tree.

The neck itself must be inspected for evidence of external damage to, or lateral displacement of, the larynx or trachea. Particular care must be taken in examination of the head and neck to avoid further cord insult by improper manipulation. Subcutaneous emphysema in the neck or supraclavicular fossa (crunch) may indicate either tracheal disruption or pneumothorax. Distended neck veins may suggest significant pericardial effusion.

Examination of the chest cavity must be meticulous. Asymmetry of expansion may be secondary to unilateral diaphragmatic paralysis, pneumothorax, multiple rib fractures with flail chest, pleural effusion (hemo/hydropneumothorax), or obstruction of a major bronchus.

Rib fractures will not be subjectively sensed as pain or tenderness by the quadriplegic, and rib-by-rib palpation for evidence of fractures should be undertaken. Open wounds to the chest wall should alert the physician to the possibility of hemothorax, pneumothorax, or tension pneumothorax. Auscultation should be carried out in an equally painstaking way with attention to symmetry of aeration.

The presence of diffuse rales suggests pulmonary edema of either cardiogenic (heart dysfunction of iatrogenic fluid overload) or noncardiogenic (acute respiratory distress syndrome, or ARDS) origin.[20, 31] Lung contusion must be considered if rales are localized or beneath an area of traumatized chest wall. Coarse rhonchi indicate retained airway secretions including blood or vomitus. Physical examination may be limited by lack of access to the posterior chest of the patient until the C-spine has been stabilized.

Chest and abdominal x-ray films should be done routinely as well as C-spine radiographs, tomograms, and computerized tomograms when indicated. Radiographic studies of ribs and long bones should be ordered according to the historical and physical findings.

INITIAL RESPIRATORY CARE

The patient should be maintained in the supine position, with positioning to decubitus and partial prone positions intermittently performed to clear secretions. Use of a turning bed (Roto-bed®) allows for this with greater ease.[35]

Humidified inspired air or oxygen keeps secretions moist and easier to mobilize.

Suctioning by trained personnel may be performed via the nasal or oral routes to clear centralized secretions in the setting of poorly effective cough.

Early insertion of a nasogastric tube for drainage of the

stomach contents will decrease the likelihood of aspiration. Decompression of gastric and intestinal distention secondary to neurogenic ileus will also facilitate diaphragmatic function.[8, 33]

Immediate attention should be directed to sequelae of thoracic trauma. Significant pleural effusions should be evaluated,[8] pneumothoraces expanded, and flail ribs or sterna stabilized.

INTUBATION

Among the earliest decisions to be made by the physician is whether intubation with assisted ventilation is necessary. Of 188 patients with acute traumatic quadriplegia seen over ten years at one center, half were found to have severe respiratory insufficiency requiring intubation.[17] Risk factors contributing to respiratory insufficiency included head trauma with coma, chest trauma, multiple fractures with hypovolemic shock, preexisting cardiac disease, and preexisting bronchopulmonary disease. Patients with complete versus incomplete cord lesions had nearly double the incidence of respiratory insufficiency of those with incomplete lesions. Advancing age was a negative prognostic factor as well.[23]

Pulmonary function must be rapidly and repeatedly assessed for immediate decisions as well as for establishing baseline values. Vital capacity, PI_{max}, PE_{max}, and arterial blood gas analysis can be measured with little disruption to simultaneous definitive care.[27]

Deterioration on serial determinations suggests that ventilatory insufficiency is imminent.

Profound hypoxemia ($PO_2 < 50$) or severe hypercapnea ($PCO_2 > 50$) will usually correlate with clinical signs and symptoms of acute respiratory distress. In such cases intubation should be undertaken immediately. Similarly, patients with extreme multiple trauma, obtundation, shock, thoracic trauma, evidence of gastric aspiration, or head and neck injuries with upper airway compromise should be intubated. Patients will often require surgery and require intubation after initial stabilization of vital signs.

If intubation is necessary, it cannot be done in the usual fashion with the neck hyperextended; it may be attempted in the neutral position via blind nasotracheal intubation. The endotracheal tube may be also passed over the flexible bronchoscope under direct visualization via the oral route. The tube should be of large internal diameter (No. 8—8 mm or larger). This will facilitate suctioning, allow passage of a flexible bronchoscope, and minimize the additional resistance of an airway smaller than the patient's own trachea.

SUCTIONING

It has been observed in quadriplegic patients that disconnection from the ventilator may result in almost immediate profound bradycardia.[4] This response is consistent within a given patient and is prevented by hyperventilation and superoxygenation or by administration of atropine or use of special suction adaptors that permit continuous pressure and oxygen administration during suctioning are other alternatives.[6]

While such a response is seen in nonquadriplegic patients as well, it may be particularly dangerous in this group.

MECHANICAL VENTILATION

Once intubated, the patient should be placed on a volume-cycled ventilator. Initial settings should include a tidal volume calculated as 10 to 12 ml/per kilogram of body weight. The FIO_2 should be adjusted to maintain a Pa_{O_2} of 70 to 75 mm Hg and the respiratory rate to achieve a Pa_{CO_2} of 40 to 45 mm Hg. The routine use of "physiologic PEEP" (positive end expiratory pressure) remains controversial; it is purported to assure inflation of small airways and prevent microatelectasis.

Addition of PEEP carries the potential risks of decreased cardiac output, direct organ toxicity (e.g., renal, hepatic) and pulmonary barotrauma (e.g., pneumothorax). It should be instituted with the assistance of a pulmonary specialist and most often with a Swan-Ganz catheter in place. More detailed review of such management is beyond the scope of this text.[5, 38]

The patient on a respirator must be protected from the most common toxicities of ventilator assistance. Twenty percent of patients requiring ventilatory assistance will have gastrointestinal tract bleeding requiring transfusion of two or more units of blood[18]; prophylactic cimetidine, ranitidine, antacids, or both should be used. Mylanta® or Maalox® should alternate with Amphojel® to avoid both diarrhea and hypophosphatemia.

Iatrogenic hyperventilation results from excessively high assisted minute ventilation. The sequelae of long-term hypocarbia include decreased cerebral blood flow and tissue oxygenation, depletion of bicarbonate and inorganic phosphate stores, and bronchoconstriction.[25] Downward adjustment of set respiratory rate is preferred to smaller tidal volumes; in this way secretion retention and atelectasis will be avoided.

ACUTE RESPIRATORY DETERIORATION

Acute respiratory deterioration in the quadriplegic patient is most often secondary to inability to adequately clear tracheobronchial secretions. This is true for patients with acute as well as stable conditions whether or not they are receiving ventilatory assistance. The deterioration is most often clinically apparent and is measurable by blood gas determination and pulmonary function testing (PFT).

Associated radiologic findings may include loss of volume with atelectasis, either discoid or major. Segmental or lobar collapse, elevation of a hemidiaphragm, or shift of mediastinal structures or trachea to the area of atelectasis will be indicative of such loss of functional lung.

Such findings in the acute stage will usually require intubation with assisted mechanical ventilation. The high tidal volume delivered by the respirator will serve to correct ventilatory insufficiency and assist in secretion mobilization.

Segmental or lobar atelectasis secondary to mucoid impaction may be cleared by the above measures. Addition of a nebulized mucolytic agent may be attempted in such a setting. Mucomyst® at a final concentration of 5% may be given up to every six hours. Because of its potential to cause broncho-spasm, it is often given in combination with nebulized bronchodilator, e.g.:

1.5cc Mucomyst® 10% + Bronkosol® 0.5 cc + 1 cc NS *OR*
1.5 cc Mucomyst® 10% + Alupent® 0.3 cc + 1 cc NS

Mucolytics should not be used in the unintubated patient with markedly impaired cough because of the increase in volume of secretions and possible "drowning."

In the intubated patient, deep tracheal suctioning combined with directed chest physical therapy may result in resolution of mucoid impaction. It must be recalled that the anatomy of the lower tracheobronchial tree allows the straight suction catheter to be effective only in the trachea and right lower lobe. Failure to clear secretions from other areas may necessitate directed suctioning with a curved-tip catheter. Most often, though, the flexible fiberoptic bronchoscope of large diameter with a large suctioning channel can be used to direct suctioning under direct visualization. Lavage and irrigation of obstructed areas is possible under such circumstances; mucolytic agents may be added if saline lavage and suction are not successful in removal of plugs.

The incidence of acute secretion-related respiratory compromise will usually decrease over time; spinal cord stability will allow for more frequent changes in position of the patient and more aggressive chest physical therapy. Evolution of abdominal wall and intercostal muscular spasticity will strengthen the patient's spontaneous cough while allowing for ventilation in the sitting or semierect (tilt board) positions.

Once the patient's ventilatory status has stabilized the management of retained secretions becomes more elective. Adequate gas exchange may allow for noninvasive management. Frequent assisted cough maneuvers may help in raising secretions,[22] at least to the level of the upper airway/oropharynx, allowing for less traumatic suctioning. The patient with a permanent tracheostomy or button may be at an advantage under such circumstances since deeper suctioning may be more feasible. As mentioned, mucolytic agents should not be used as a rule in patients who cannot be frequently and reliably suctioned.

A defined period should be allowed for resolution of such major atelectasis/secretion retention. The temptation to tolerate major volume loss in a setting of adequate gas exchange should be avoided. Long-term secretion retention may result in bronchiectasis with subsequent chronic secretion production, repeated infection, and bronchospasm. Permanent loss of function of major lung segments is obviously not desirable in patients with permanent severe restrictive disease already present on a neuromuscular basis.

Antihistamines, excessive diuresis, and other pharmacologic interventions likely to result in dry secretions should be avoided. Similarly, early aggressive management of respiratory infection with humidification and chest physical therapy maneuvers (see below) will help prevent atelectatic episodes.

OTHER CAUSES OF EARLY RESPIRATORY COMPROMISE

The acute respiratory distress syndrome (ARDS) or noncardiogenic pulmonary edema has recently been recognized as a potential complication of acute spinal cord injury.[28, 32] Originally described in association with intracranial catastrophes including trauma, intracranial bleeding, and seizures,[1] it is believed that injury to the CNS may result in a massive outpouring of sympathetic catecholamines. Whether it is a sudden rise in peripheral vascular resistance that precipitates acute heart failure or whether the primary disorder is at the pulmonary vascular level mediated by histamine and other vasoactive substances is unknown. The sudden appearance of acute hypoxemia with auscultatory evidence of pulmonary edema has been observed repeatedly within the first 24 hours following spinal cord injury in which no thoracic trauma is present.

Physical examination may be typical of left heart failure, with the appearance of rales, wheezes, and neck venous distention, or may be relatively unrevealing. Impaired respiratory excursion may obscure the presence of alveolar fluid and rales. A chest roentgenogram will usually reveal pulmonary vascular congestion. Such findings in the absence of cardiomegaly should suggest ARDS.[20, 31]

The absence of elevated left heart filling pressures, as determined by Swan-Ganz catheterization, classically differentiates cardiogenic from noncardiogenic pulmonary edema.[38]

In cases where chest trauma has occurred, cardiac tamponade should also be considered and will similarly be excluded by Swan-Ganz measurements.

Intubation with supportive ventilatory assistance must be instituted immediately. If blood pressure allows, a trial of diuretic therapy may be undertaken until a Swan-Gatz catheter is placed for measurement of intravascular volume.

The possibility of such a complication mandates judicious fluid resuscitation in "spinal shock."[28] The hypotension commonly seen in the acute phases of cervical spinal cord injury is likely secondary to decreased sympathetic vasomotor tone and decreased peripheral vascular resistance. Expansion of the vascular space in acute quadriplegia allows for accommodation of large volumes of infused fluid without increasing central venous pressure (CVF). The observed rise in total peripheral resistance within a day or two of injury may trigger acute volume overload and pulmonary edema. Early hypotension is best treated with pharmacologic support rather than overly vigorous fluid replacement so as to avoid cardiogenic pulmonary edema or to minimize severity of noncardiogenic edema with respiratory failure.

Pancreatitis has been described as complicating acute spinal cord injury even in the absence of abdominal trauma.[7] Decreased sympathetic tone with altered neurocontrol of the sphincter of Oddi, alterations of blood flow to the pancreas, as well as use of opiates and steroids may each cause pancreatitis. The relationship of pancreatitis to ARDS has been well described and is postulated as secondary to complement activation by release of pancreatic enzymes.[20, 30] The absence of abdominal pain in acute quadriplegia as is normally seen in pancreatitis makes routine measurement of serum amylase levels important in respiratory management of quadriplegics as a predictor of potential respiratory failure.

Aspiration of gastric contents may occur in acute quadriplegia in the presence or absence of abdominal trauma or coma. Gastric contents of pH less than 2.5 and/or presence of food particles will predispose to acute respiratory distress syndrome as described above.[39]

Fat emboli must be suspected in cases of trauma to long bones, particularly the femoral and tibial shafts. It has been shown that at the time of the injury, fat microglobules enter the venous circulation from the marrow and surrounding fatty tissues and migrate to the lungs where some are deposited. Others continue through to the brain, kidneys, skin, and other organs. The microglobules entrapped in the pulmonary circulation are hydrolyzed by the lipoprotein lipase into free fatty acids. Release of fat thromboplastin may initiate intravascular coagulation with resulting fibrin deposition and platelet aggregation. In combination, the pathways may result in diffuse pulmonary capillary damage with ARDS.[1, 20]

The classic occurrence of fat-embolus-related disease is at 24 to 48 hours postinjury and presents as irritability, headache, and neurologic deterioration in association with tachypnea and poor blood gases. It must be emphasized that long bone trauma per se need not be present, and that the time course can be variable.

Sepsis is thought to be the most significant factor in development of ARDS. Patients with multiple trauma, bladder catheters, IVs, and/or steroids must be carefully observed with a high index of suspicion.[20, 31]

BLOOD TRANSFUSIONS

Traumatized patients with hemorrhage may receive large numbers of blood transfusions. Platelet and fibrin aggregates microemboli may become trapped in pulmonary capillaries. Transfused leukocytes may become similarly lodged in pulmonary capillaries. In either case, vasoactive substances and/or complement may result in damage to alveolar-capillary membrane with ARDS.[28] This is usually rapidly reversing following the completion of transfusion.[12]

SLEEP APNEA

Early in the course of spinal cord injury, the level of the lesion may ascend or descend by several segments via evolution of a cone of edema or hemorrhage. Thus, a low C-spine injury may evolve to further damage diaphragmatic activity that may have been normal shortly after injury.

If the cone extends to involve the anterolateral portion of the cord in the C-2 C-4 area, sleep apnea may occur. It has been observed in percutaneous cordotomy that the greatest risk is seen within the first five nights following cord injury.[32]

UNILATERAL DIAPHRAGMATIC PARALYSIS

Approximately 2% of traumatic quadriplegic patients seen at one center over a 20-year period were found to have unilateral diaphragmatic paralysis.[9] Paralysis may have been a result of gunshot or closed wound to the cervical spine or secondary to direct trauma to the chest or abdomen resulting in diaphragmatic rupture. Right and left hemidiaphragms were affected with similar frequency.

Of note is that, in most cases reviewed, the paralysis was transient, with reversal in approximately 2.5 months. An ascending swelling of the cord above the level of injury, stretching of the phrenic nerve, and other mechanisms have been proposed for such transient dysfunction of nerves arising from C-4 as well as C-3 and C-5. In most circumstances, no specific therapy is instituted. Overall improvement in pulmonary function may reflect diaphragmatic motion.

CHEST PHYSICAL THERAPY

The patient's acute and long-term respiratory status will be benefited by chest physical therapy in combination with the numerous respiratory therapy modalities reviewed.

Chest physical therapy is a series of manipulative devices designed to prevent pulmonary complications and to improve airway function in acute and chronic pulmonary disease.[36] Bronchial hygiene may be assisted by IPPB, postural drainage, percussion and vibration, and assisted cough.

POSTURAL DRAINAGE

Postural drainage utilizes the principle that secretion drainage is facilitated by body positions that allow mucus to flow in the direction of gravity.[36] Because ventilatory function in acute quadriplegic patients is better in the supine than in the upright position, regular expansion and drainage of basal and posterior lung segments will thus be infrequent and at a disadvantage. Intermittent drainage of these areas by postural drainage under the direct supervision of a skilled therapist may be safely achieved. Continuously rotating beds have been developed to facilitate frequent changes in position in the acute setting.[35] The addition of chest percussion, or clapping of a cupped hand against the chest wall, will assist in loosening peripheral and adherent mucus secretions. Chest vibration during exhalation may be performed as well.

Assisted cough[22] is a maneuver whereby manual compression of flaccid abdominal musculature at end-inspiration will increase intra-abdominal pressure during the compressive and expulsive phases of cough.

All of these modalities may be used in combination in the acute and convalescent phases of spinal cord injury. Patients and families may be instructed in simple positioning for postural drainage and in assisted cough technique following hospital discharge. They may be prescribed for daily use in patients with underlying chronic secretion problems (e.g., chronic bronchitis) or recommended for institution at the first suggestion of an acute respiratory infection.

INCENTIVE SPIROMETRY

The incentive spirometer was initially developed as an operant conditioning device to encourage sustained deep breathing in the rehabilitation of quadriplegics.[10] It has since been used routinely to prevent atelectasis and to facilitate clearance of pulmonary secretions in clinical situations where the patient would otherwise favor a respiratory pattern of shallow tidal volumes, e.g., following thoracic or abdominal surgery. It may be used in the stable quadriplegic for such purposes as well. It is easily used without the assistance of trained respiratory or nursing personnel and may be used many times during the day, both in the hospital and at home.

It has been observed that sudden decreases in the ability to achieve the expected or usual level may be the first suggestion of impending pneumonia or atelectasis.[36] In such an event, or in other acute situations where inability to achieve adequate levels of inspiration occur to assure proper bronchial hygiene, IPPB may be substituted.

INTERMITTENT POSITIVE PRESSURE BREATHING (IPPB)

"The principle is that of repeated administration of a series of passive inhalations of variable volumes delivered by a pressure-cycled respirator, each followed by the subject exhaling into the ambient atmosphere. The machine is triggered by the patient's inspiratory effort. The device may be used via oral mouthpiece or face mask or it may be attached to a tracheotomy tube. The tidal volume is achieved via pressure settings."[39]

The advantages over the incentive spirometer include the following: (1) the ability to deliver a tidal volume greater than the patient's own tidal volume; (2) a minimal inspiratory effort is needed to "trigger" a machine breath; (3) patient fatigue and poor endurance are less of a limiting factor; and (4) humidification and medication can be delivered. Desirable results include mobilization of secretions, decrease in work of breathing, improved gas exchange, relief of atelectasis, and humidification of the airway. Needless to say, concomitant chest physical therapy including postural drainage and assisted cough may be necessary to clear the secretions mobilized by the IPPB machine.

IPPB therapy, however, carries risks associated with positive pressure ventilators, including pulmonary barotrauma and circulatory embarrassment. Direct supervision by trained personnel is required for each session although families may be taught to administer IPPB therapy.

RESPIRATORY REHABILITATION

Simple respiratory repetitive exercises can be undertaken with uncomplicated machinery. These can be done at the bedside and continued at home. Early progression from ventilator dependence to independence may be achieved. Prevention of serious respiratory infections may result over the long term.

Frog breathing or glossopharyngeal breathing, described by Montero et al. in 1967,[29] involves inflating the lungs by use of intact muscles of the mouth, pharynx, and larynx as a respiratory pump. Chronic quadriplegics could be taught within several weeks to add up to 1 L of air to baseline vital capacity by ten to 20 glossopharyngeal gulps. Gulping continues until considerable pressure is felt in the throat and upper chest; air is then expelled with secretions removed as a functional cough. Repetition of such exercise is demonstrated to improve MBC, VC, and maximal expiratory flow significantly. Glossopharyngeal breathing appears to function as a sigh with increase in lung volume to full vital capacity. The lung and thoracic cage compliances are at better advantage for effective cough and clearing of secretions.

Measures aimed directly at true rehabilitation of respiratory muscles, as opposed to modifying respiratory pattern, emphasize the concept of multiple repetitions at increasing loads. The principle of operant conditioning combined with use of a graduated incentive spirometer was described in 1977.[10, 11] Various inspiratory goals are set to correspond to increasing vital capacities. The patient's recognition of increasing muscle strength following repeated exercise repetition is the reward and impetus for continued exercise. All patients studied over six to 12 weeks showed marked improvement in FVC. This was true in patients with old or new cervical lesions and was independent of earlier ventilator assistance requirements.

It has been demonstrated more recently[15] that inspiratory muscle fatigue occurs in quadriplegics with very little extra respiratory load compared to normal subjects. Since only diaphragm and sternocleidomastoid were operant for inspiration, alternation with intercostal muscles cannot take place in fatiguing situations as would occur in normal persons. An *inspi-*

ratory resistive breathing training program utilizing a simple Rudolph valve has been devised to train ventilatory muscle endurance. Two 15-minute sessions daily for eight weeks resulted in a significant increase in both diaphragmatic muscle strength and endurance. Less subjective respiratory fatigue was present as well.[15]

LONG-TERM CARE

The long-term goal for the physician is to achieve a state of optimal respiratory stability for the remainder of the patient's life. Ideally, the patient will not require chronic ventilatory assistance or artificial airway. Prevention of bronchopulmonary infection with possible respiratory (gas-exchange) embarrassment is to be sought whether or not assisted ventilation is needed.

The physician must therefore outline a program for the patient which may include the following facts:
- Assessing need for long-term ventilatory assistance[19]
- Type of artificial airway
- Care of artificial airway
- Respiratory care/patient toilet during chronic maintenance status and in event of acute respiratory/other medical decompensation
- Measures to improve respiratory function
- Pharmacologic intervention
- Measures to prevent and control respiratory infection
- Avoidance of tobacco and alcohol which will suppress ciliary clearance mechanisms

TRACHEOSTOMY

The serial measurement of pulmonary function, as stated previously, begins early in the care of the acute quadriplegic.[27] Just as the need for acute endotracheal intubation is determined by both measured pulmonary function and clinical evaluation, so is the assessment of need for tracheostomy. Tracheostomy may be required in order to allow for certain neurosurgical or maxillofacial surgical procedures directly related to the cause of acute traumatic quadriplegia. More classically, however, tracheostomy is mandated when mechanical ventilation is needed for more than seven to 14 days. Nasotracheal/orotracheal tubes are potentially damaging to the subglottic region beyond this period. The presence of the ET tube and low-pressure cuff will potentially result in subglottic stenosis and must be replaced by an electively placed tracheostomy tube. Patient discomfort caused by the former tube is usually relieved by creation of a tracheostomy as well. The frequently encountered hesitation to perform this "extra procedure" with implication of prolonged ventilatory dependence is not appropriate; once the tracheostomy tube is no longer needed, the stoma, if properly cared for, will spontaneously seal within days. Premature ventilator removal prompted by the desire to "extubate" is not infrequently followed by acute respiratory decompensation requiring reintubation.

TRACHEOSTOMY BUTTON

Once it has been established that the patient no longer needs regular ventilatory assistance or suctioning, the tracheostomy tube may be removed. It is, however, desirable to maintain easy airway access, particularly in high quadriplegics in whom the newly achieved baseline does not provide significant reserve in case of acute respiratory decompensation, e.g., pneumonia. Various plastic and Teflon® prostheses may be fitted to the stoma size and inserted. They may remain in place indefinitely with minimal care. The purpose of the button is to maintain stoma patency in case of acute decompensation, at which time it is replaced by a tracheostomy tube. It is not designed for ventilator attachment or for frequent suctioning.[36]

LONG-TERM VENTILATORY ASSISTANCE

The quadriplegic patient whose condition has stabilized medically but who remains dependent on ventilatory support is necessarily limited in rehabilitation potential. Numerous assistive devices are available that are relatively portable, that is, do not require an ICU setting for use.

Pressure- or volume-cycled ventilators are presently available that are of typewriter size. They are AC and battery powered, alarmed, reliable, and easily fit under an electric wheelchair.[8]

The volume ventilators are most reliable in tidal volume settings and are presently available with sigh mechanisms.

Patients with tracheostomy tubes may use such assistive devices continuously, intermittently throughout the day, or nightly only. Such assistance may be only required in the event of respiratory infection or other intercurrent medical problem.

External devices include the cuirass and Pneumobelt, which provide external compression to the chest or abdomen and may be useful in patients without tracheostomies.[36] The alteration in usual muscular relationships caused by chest wall spasticity and abdominal flaccidity make this less useful a modality than ventilators per se in quadriplegic respiratory failure.

PHRENIC NERVE STIMULATION

In the 1960s, phrenic nerve stimulation (PNS) to pace the diaphragm was first applied to patients with acute and chronic ventilatory failure. Initial success was met with alternate hemidiaphragmatic pacing at rates of 12 to 15 breaths per minute for up to 60% of the day. Poor long-term adequacy of such a regimen has resulted in more recent experience with uninterrupted simultaneous pacing of both hemidiaphragms using low-frequency stimulation at respiratory rates of five to nine per minute.[13]

More current techniques allow for improved pulmonary function and minute volumes, better air mixing, less myopathic change in the diaphragm, and less diaphragmatic fatigue. Minute volume has been noted to improve for a given pacing rate at one year's time, suggesting an exercise/conditioning effect of the diaphragm muscle by the regular paced contractures.[14]

It is recommended that this technique be reserved for patients with a high cervical lesion who are neurologically stable and with otherwise good rehabilitation potential.

Because of coincidental acute medical problems encountered early in the course of quadriplegic ventilatory insufficiency, and because of the unpredictability of recovery at the time of injury, it is recommended that two to three months elapse before considering PNS.[8]

The status of the phrenic nerves and diaphragm must be investigated; voluntary diaphragmatic control can be quantitated fluoroscopically. Excursion of each hemidiaphragm in centimeters is measured from end-expiration to full inspiration on the fluoroscope screen. The status of the phrenic nerve is assessed by transcutaneous phrenic nerve stimulation, the application of impulses to the phrenic nerve by use of an electrode probe placed on the skin of the neck overlaying the nerve. A hiccup-like contraction of the hemidiaphragm will be visible at the costal insertion of the muscle; the strength of the contraction will estimate partial to full intactness of the lower motor neuron.[13]

CONCLUSION

A respiratory therapy regimen must be individualized for each patient both acutely and on a long-term basis. Some patients may do well very shortly after spinal cord injury and have few pulmonary complications. Regular use of incentive spirometry will both improve respiratory function and endurance and minimize the likelihood of bronchopulmonary infection. Training the family in postural drainage and assisted cough with an available IPPB machine in event of respiratory infection will avoid serious deterioration in gas exchange and bronchial hygiene.

Recent physiologic and clinical understanding of respiratory and clinical aspects of quadriplegia hopefully will allow the promise that these painstaking routines and efforts will result in meaningful longevity.

REFERENCES

1. Amato J.J., Rheinlander H.F., Cleveland R.J.: Post-traumatic adult respiratory distress syndrome. *Ortho. Clin. North Am.* 9:693–713, 1978.
2. Bake B., Fugl-Meyer A.R., Grumby G.: Breathing patterns and re-

gional ventilation distribution in tetraplegic patients and in normal subjects. *Clin. Sci.* 42:117–128, 1972.

3. Bergofsky E.H.: Respiratory failure in disorders of the thoracic cage. *Am. Rev. Respir. Dis.* 119:643–669, 1979.

4. Berk J.L., Levy M.N.: Profound reflex bradycardia produced by transient hypoxemia or hypercapnia in man. *Eur. Surg. Res.* 9:75–84, 1977.

5. Boysen P.G.: Hemodynamic monitoring in the adult respiratory distress syndrome. *Clin. Chest Med.* 3:157–169, 1982.

6. Cabal L., Devaskar S., Siassi B., et al.: New endotracheal tube adaptor reducing cardiopulmonary effects of suctioning. *Crit. Care Med.* 7:552–555, 1979.

7. Carey M.E., Nance F.C., Kirgis H.D., et al.: Pancreatitis following spinal cord injury. *J. Neurosurg.* 47:917–22, 1977.

8. Carter R.E.: Medical management of pulmonary complications of spinal cord injury. *Adv. Neurol.* 22:261–269, 1979.

9. Carter R.E.: Unilateral diaphragmatic paralysis in spinal cord injury patients. *Paraplegia* 18:267–273, 1980.

10. Cheshire D.J.E., Flack W.J.: The use of operant conditioning techniques in the respiratory rehabilitation of the tetraplegic. *Paraplegia* 16:162–174, 1978.

11. Corson J.A., Grant J.L., Moulton D.P., et al.: Use of biofeedback in weaning paralyzed patients from respirators. *Chest* 76:543–545, 1979.

12. Divertie M.B.: Diffuse alveolar damage, respiratory failure, and blood transfusion. *Mayo Clin. Proc.* 59:643–644, 1984.

13. Glenn W.W.L., Hogan J.F., Phelps M.L.: Ventilatory support of the quadriplegic patient with respiratory paralysis by diaphragm pacing. *Surg. Clin. North Am.* 60:1055–1078, 1980.

14. Glenn W.W.L., Hogan J.F., Loke J.S.O. et al.: Ventilatory support by pacing of the conditioned diaphragm in quadriplegia. *N. Engl. J. Med.* 310:1150–1155, 1984.

15. Gross D., Ladd H.W., Riley E.J., et al.: The effect of training on strength and endurance of the diaphragm in quadriplegia. *Am. J. Med.* 68:27–35, 1980.

16. Haas F., Pineda H., Axen K., et al.: Time related, posturally induced changes in pulmonary function in spinal cord injured man. *Am. Rev. Resp. Dis.* 117:344A, 1978.

17. Hachen H.J.: Idealized care of the acutely injured spinal cord in Switzerland. *J. Trauma* 17:931–936, 1977.

18. Harris S.K., Bone R.C., Ruth W.E.: Gastrointestinal hemorrhage in

patients in a respiratory intensive care unit. *Chest* 72:301–304, 1972.

19. Hodgkin J.D., Bowser M.A., Burton G.G.: Respiratory weaning. *Crit. Care Med.* 2:96–102, 1974.
20. Hudson L.D.: Causes of the adult respiratory distress syndrome—clinical recognition. *Clin. Chest Med.* 3:195–212, 1982.
21. Irwin R.S., Rosen M.J., Braman S.S.: Cough: A comprehensive review. *Arch. Intern. Med.* 137:1186–1191, 1977.
22. Kirby M.A., Barnieras M.J., Siebens A.A.: An evaluation of assisted cough in quadriparetic patients. *Arch. Phys. Med. Rehabil.* 47:705–710, 1966.
23. Kiwerski J., Weiss M., Chrostowska T.: Analysis of mortality of patients after cervical spine trauma. *Paraplegia* 19:347–351, 1981.
24. Luce J.M., Culver B.H.: Respiratory muscle function in health and disease. *Chest* 81:82–90, 1982.
25. Mazzara J.T., Ayres S.M., Grace W.J.: Extreme hypocapnia in the critically ill patient. *Am. J. Med.* 56:450–456, 1974.
26. McKinley A.C., Auchincloss J.H. Jr., Gilbert R., et al.: Pulmonary function, ventilatory control, and respiratory complications in quadriplegic subjects. *Am. Rev. Respir. Dis.* 100:526–562, 1969.
27. McMichan J.C., Michel L., Westbrook P.R.: Pulmonary dysfunction following traumatic quadriplegia. *J.A.M.A.* 243:528–531, 1980.
28. Meyer G.A., Berman I.R., Doty D.B., et al.: Hemodynamic responses to acute quadriplegia with or without chest trauma. *J. Neurosurg.* 34:168–177, 1971.
29. Montero J.C., Feldman D.J., Montero D.: Effects of glossopharyngeal breathing on respiratory function after cervical cord transection. *Arch. Phys. Med. Rehabil.* 48:650–663, 1967.
30. Murphy B., Pack A.I., Imrie C.W.: The mechanisms of arterial hypoxia occurring in acute pancreatitis. *Q. J. Med.* 49:151–163, 1980.
31. Petty T.L.: Adult respiratory distress syndrome. *Semin. Respir. Med.* 3:219–224, 1982.
32. Poe R.H., Reisman J.L., Rodenhouse T.G.: Pulmonary edema in cervical spinal cord injury. *J. Trauma* 18:71–73, 1978.
33. Quimby C.W. Jr., Williams R.N., Greifenstein F.E.: Anesthetic problems of the acute quadriplegic patient. *Anesth. Analg.* 52:333–340, 1973.
34. Roncoroni A.J.: Lack of breathlessness during apnea in a patient with high spinal cord transection. *Chest* 62:514–515, 1972.

35. Schimmel L., Civetta J.N., Kirby R.R.: A new mechanical method to influence pulmonary perfusion in critically ill patients. *Crit. Care Med.* 5:277–278, 1977.
36. Shapiro B.A., Harrison R.A., Trout C.A.: *Clinical Application of Respiratory Care.* Chicago, Year Book Medical Publishers, 1979.
37. Silver J.F., Lehr R.P.: Dyspnea during generalized spasms in tetraplegic patients. *J. Neurol., Neurosurg. Psychiatry.* 44:842–845, 1981.
38. Wood L.D.H., Prewitt R.M.: Cardiovascular management in acute hypoxemic respiratory failure. *Am. J. Cardiol.* 47:963–972, 1981.
39. Wynne J.W.: Aspiration pneumonitis: Correlation of experimental models with clinical disease. *Clin. Chest Med.* 3:25–34, 1982.
39. Ziment I.: Intermittent positive pressure breathing, in Burton G.G., Gee G.N., Hodgkin J.E. (eds.): *Respiratory Care: A Guide to Clinical Practice.* Philadelphia, J.B. Lippincott Co., 1977, pp. 457–500.

4

Pneumonia

ROBERT A. PRESS, M.D., PH.D.

SCOPE OF THE PROBLEM

PNEUMONIA IS an extremely common infection in spinal cord injury patients. Such patients often have paralyzed intercostal and accessory muscles and have poor cough reflexes. Therefore, they have difficulty clearing their secretions and are prone to both aspiration and pyogenic bacterial pneumonias Frequent mucus plugging contributes to their susceptibility to infection distal to the obstructed bronchial segment. Good pulmonary toilet is therefore critical in this group, and can lead to a dramatic decrease in the incidence of pulmonary infection.

DIAGNOSIS OF PNEUMONIA

Diagnosis is, as always, dependent upon history, physical examination, and laboratory data. If the patient is observed to vomit, with gastric contents suctioned from the tracheobronchial tree and a new infiltrate appearing immediately thereafter on chest x-ray, the diagnosis of aspiration pneumonia is certainly straightforward. However, the situation is often not so clear-cut, and in fact infection may at times be difficult to distinguish from atelectasis, pulmonary infarction, or even pulmonary edema.

The presence of fever, signs of consolidation on physical examination, and an infiltrate on chest x-ray are all suggestive, but certainly not pathognomonic, of pneumonia. The additional finding of an elevated white blood cell (WBC) count, especially with a shift to the left, is helpful. However, most impressive for the diagnosis of aspiration or suppurative bacterial pneumonia is the presence of purulent sputum.

In assessing the etiology of pneumonia, the sputum Gram's stain is critical, and in fact probably more important in some respects than the sputum culture. The Gram's stain supplies two pieces of information not available from the culture: (1) the degree of inflammation present, i.e., number of polys, and (2) the predominant organism in the sputum. This second point cannot be overemphasized. The gram stain provides information regarding the proportion of various types of organisms, and answers the question, "Is there a predominant organism and, if so, what type is it (i.e., gram-positive cocci in pairs, gram-negative rods, etc.)?" On culture, however, certain organisms will grow much faster than others, so that a gram-negative rod initially present in small quantity might completely overgrow a more fastidious gram-positive coccus. It is not at all unusual, for example, for a Gram's stain to show sheets of lancet-shaped gram-positive diplococci, but for the culture to fail to grow *Pneumococcus,* since this organism may at times be difficult to isolate.

If the patient is not intubated and it is not possible to obtain a good coughed sputum sample (with polys present on Gram's stain), nasotracheal, transtracheal, or bronchoscopic aspiration should be used to obtain a sample.

If the patient has fever, an infiltrate, and a pleural effusion, the effusion should be tapped, with the fluid so obtained also gram-stained and sent for culture as well as chemistries and cell count with differential.

SPECIFIC PNEUMONIAS AND THEIR TREATMENT

Before considering specific pneumonic infections, a few general comments should be made regarding therapy. Antibiotics are certainly one therapeutic modality in the treatment of pneumonia in the spinal cord injury patient. However, if used alone they will often fail to eradicate the infection. Good pulmonary toilet is especially critical in the successful treatment of this group of patients, as is adequate ventilation. To achieve these two goals (toilet and ventilation), tracheal intubation may at times be necessary, sometimes with mechanical ventilation.

Naturally, the spinal cord injury patient may contract all types of pneumonia to which the general population is susceptible, including viral, myoplasma, and chlamydial, as well as bacterial. However, there are certain lung infections to which this patient is more susceptible than is the general population, and these will be considered here. They can roughly be divided into aspiration pneumonia, gram-positive pyogenic pneumonias, and gram-negative pyogenic pneumonias.

ASPIRATION PNEUMONIA

Many spinal cord injury patients develop gastric dilatation secondary to air-swallowing and subsequently regurgitate gastric contents.[1] This, coupled with their poor cough reflex, makes them subject to repeated episodes of aspiration. The resulting pneumonia occurs in a dependent portion of the lung. If the patient is recumbent, the posterior segments of the upper lobes and the superior segments of the lower lobes are dependent. Right-sided infection predominates due to the angle of the right mainstem bronchus. If the patient is upright at the time of aspiration, pneumonia will likely occur in the basilar segments of the lower lobes.

Many episodes of aspiration of gastric contents result in a straightforward chemical pneumonitis. Fever and infiltrate on chest x-ray both appear within a matter of hours after the event and often disappear within a matter of days. Sputum may show polys and few organisms on Gram's stain. What occurs in this case is essentially a chemical burn. Although such damaged lung tissue is quite susceptible to bacterial infection, there is no role for prophylactic antibiotics in this situation.[2] They will only serve to select out resistant organisms, should an infection ensue. The role of steroids in aspiration is still somewhat controversial. If they are used, they should be begun as soon as possible after the event (probably within minutes), should be used in high dosage (approximately 2 gm of methylprednisolone per day), and should be continued for a maximum of two days.

Bacterial aspiration pneumonia can and does certainly occur in this patient group. In general, the bacteria aspirated are those in the mouth and upper airways. In a nonhospitalized patient, these are primarily penicillin-sensitive anaerobes (e.g., *Peptostreptococcus, Bacteroides melaninogenicus,* and *Fusobacterium nucleatum*) and aerobic gram-positive cocci (e.g., *Streptococcus viridans* and *Pneumococcus*). Gram's stain of the sputum in this situation shows many polys and mixed flora, with no predominant organism present. Sputum culture shows "normal flora." Such a pneumonia may be treated with low-dose penicillin (2 to 3 million units/day). Even when *Bacteroides fragilis,* a penicillin-resistant anaerobe, is present, this mixed infection usually responds to penicillin. An excellent alternative drug, especially if the patient fails to defervesce within 3 to 5 days, is clindamycin.

Many spinal cord injury patients have been hospitalized for long periods of time, and some have received multiple courses of antibiotics. The bacteria that colonize the mouth and upper airways in such patients are different from those in the outpatient community. There is a higher proportion of *Staphylococcus aureus,* and a much higher proportion of aerobic gram-negative rods colonizing these patients. When aspiration occurs in this situation, the resulting pneumonia may still be caused by a mixture of aerobic and anaerobic organisms, but aerobic gram-negative rods and, at times, *S. aureus* may predominate. A sputum Gram's stain and culture are critical in the final selection of antibiotic regimen. Initially, before culture results are available, clindamycin plus an aminoglycoside, or a "third-generation" cephalosporin would provide broad-spectrum coverage.

Complications of aspiration pneumonia include necrotizing pneumonia, abscess formation, and empyema. Necrotizing pneumonia should be treated with high-dose antibiotics. Initial therapy for lung abscess should also be high-dose antibiotics. After defervescence occurs, appropriate oral therapy can be substituted and continued until either the cavity disappears on x-ray, or a small stable residual lesion is present. All empyemas should be drained.[2]

PYOGENIC BACTERIAL PNEUMONIAS

Gram-Positive Cocci

Pneumococcus. Pneumococcal pneumonia, which is often lobar, classically begins suddenly with a rigor, following which fever and a cough productive of rusty sputum develop. Gram's stain of the sputum usually shows many polys with lancet-shaped gram-positive diplococci, some of which may be intracellular. The organism may be difficult to isolate on culture. It is extremely sensitive to low-dose penicillin (2.4 million units/day or less) and can be treated orally, with length of therapy generally ten days. Alternatives to penicillin in pneumococcal pneumonia are erythromycin, clindamycin cephalothin, cefazolin, cephapirin, and cephalexin. Bacteremia occurs in at least 20% to 30% of cases.

Pneumonia caused by this organism is not uncommonly complicated by metastatic foci of infection, including meninges (meningitis), heart valve(s) (endocarditis), and joints (arthritis). When metastatic foci of infection exist, the dose of penicillin must be increased.

Staphylococcus aureus. Staphylococcal pneumonia is commonly acquired in-hospital or follows influenzal infection. Diabetics are especially susceptible to infection with this organism. The pneumonia is frequently rapidly progressive, and leads to pneumatocele and/or abscess formation. Sputum Gram's stain commonly shows polys and round gram-positive cocci in clusters.

A primary S. aureus pneumonia is usually not accompanied by bacteremia, nor are metastatic foci of infection common. However, if multiple foci of staphylococcal pneumonia are present, the pneumonia may not be primary, but rather may represent metastatic foci of infection with another primary source (e.g., endocarditis), with the organism arriving in the lung via a hematogenous route.

A penicillinase-resistant penicillin like oxacillin, nafcillin, or methicillin, (2 gm every four to six hours intravenously) is usually the antimicrobial of choice for treatment, with cephalothin (2 gm every four to six hours), cefazolin (1 gm every eight hours), or cephapirin (2 gm every four to six hours) acceptable alternatives. If the strain is methicillin resistant, vancomycin (500 mg IV every six hours if renal function is normal) should be used. Length of therapy is at least two weeks.

Gram-Negative Bacilli

Hemophilus influenzae. This organism is a common cause of pneumonia in patients with chronic lung disease. Gram's stain shows polys with gram-negative pleomorphic coccobacilli. The antibiotic of choice is ampicillin or amoxicillin for susceptible strains, but in some institutions up to one third of strains are resistant to these agents. In this case, cefamandole, cefuroxime, a "third generation" cephalosporin, or chloramphenicol may be used. Length of therapy is generally two weeks.

Gram-Negative Enteric Bacilli. Included in this group are *Klebsiella pneumoniae, Escherichia coli,* and *Enterobacter* species, among others. The organisms are usually hospital acquired. Gram's stain of sputum shows polys and gram-negative bacilli. For some strains, especially *K. pneumoniae,* the bacilli are plump, with capsules obvious. The pneumonia may be necrotizing, sometimes with abscess formation.

Many authorities recommend the use of two antibiotic agents to treat these infections. The use of synergistic combinations is suggested, e.g., cephalosporin or semisynthetic penicillin plus aminoglycoside for susceptible strains. The use of aminoglycosides alone is not advisable for a serious pneumonia, since this group of antibiotics does not in general penetrate the lung parenchyma well. The length of antibiotic therapy for these infections is usually longer than for gram-positive organisms, and is commonly at least three weeks.

Pseudomonas aeruginosa. This species is almost always hospital-acquired, and is extremely common in patients on respirators. Gram's stain of the sputum shows polys and gram-negative bacilli. The rods are not usually as plump as many of the enterics. As for the gram-negative enterics, the use of a synergistic antibiotic combination is recommended, most often ticarcillin (3 gm every four hours with normal renal function) and tobramycin if the strain is sensitive. Some of the "third-generation" cephalosporins, like cefoperazone and ceftazidime, also have good antipseudomonal activity, as does imipenem.

Assessment of Therapy

In general, the patient should show clinical signs of improvement within five to seven days if he or she is on the proper therapeutic regimen. Such improvement may be evidenced by decreased fever, decreased WBC count, and thinner and decreased quantity of sputum. Resolution of infiltrates on chest x-ray may lag significantly behind clinical improvement, and in fact may take four weeks or more. However, worsening infiltrates while undergoing therapy are certainly a poor sign.

Failure of the patient to improve may be secondary to inadequate antibiotic therapy, with infection caused by a resistant organism or by multiple organisms, one or some of which may be resistant to the current antibiotic regimen. On the other hand, antibiotic therapy may be adequate, but poor pulmonary toilet may be the problem.

Sometimes most parameters point to clinical improvement, but the patient remains febrile after one week of therapy, or initially defervesces only to respike fevers after one week. In such cases, the physician must distinguish among continued infection, superinfection, and noninfectious causes of fever. Noninfectious causes for fever include drug fever, atelectasis, and, in some cases (as is common with pneumococcal pneumonia), sterile pleural effusions. If all parameters other than fever point to clinical improvement, infection is unlikely to be the cause of fever. The question of superinfection is considered in more detail below.

Colonization vs. Superinfection

The tracheobronchial trees of many, if not most patients treated for pneumonia will become colonized by organisms resistant to the antibiotic regimen utilized in the treatment. Such colonization commonly occurs about seven days into therapy. Sputum cultures begin to grow the resistant strains, and the question inevitably arises as to whether the patient is simply colonized with the new organisms, or is superinfected. The appearance of these resistant organisms is especially common in spinal cord injury patients, many of whom have undergone tracheal intubation and may require mechanical ventilation during an acute infection.

It is critical to distinguish colonization, which requires no change in antibiotic therapy, from superinfection, which does. To make this distinction, seven criteria are evaluated, with the following questions answered:

1. *Sputum Gram's stain.*—Are the polys and organisms decreasing in quantity or increasing?

2. *Chest x-ray.*—Is the infiltrate improving (or stable) or worsening?

3. *Fever.*—Is the temperature decreasing, or are fever spikes persisting or becoming higher?

4. *Respiratory signs.*—Is the patient breathing more easily, or is he (or she) having persistent or increasing difficulty (with increased tachypnea, etc)?

5. *Secretions.*—Are tracheobronchial secretions decreasing in purulence and quantity, or are they (stable or) increasing?

6. *WBC count.*— Is the WBC count back to (or approaching) normal, or has it remained high or risen again after having returned to normal?

7. *Arterial blood gases.*—Are the blood gas values improving or worsening?

If, by all of these criteria, the patient is worsening, he or she is likely superinfected, and the antibiotic regimen should be modified accordingly. If, on the other hand, all or most of these aspects are improving, the new (resistant) organisms are almost certainly simply colonizing the upper respiratory tract, and no change in therapy is required.

REFERENCES

1. Bellamy R., Pitts F.W., Stauffer E.S.: Respiratory complications in traumatic quadriplegia. *J. Neurosurg.* 39:596, 1973.
2. Bartlett J.G.: Aspiration pneumonia. *Clin. Notes Respir. Dis.,* Spring, vol. 3, 1980.

5

The Neurogenic Bladder and Voiding Dysfunction

ZAFAR KHAN, M.D.

IN VIRTUALLY ALL cases of quadriplegia, there is some degree of voiding dysfunction present. This dysfunction in turn leads to loss of voluntary voiding, which results in urinary retention with attendant infection and episodes of autonomic crisis.

The increased understanding of the neurogenic bladder and its complications has resulted in vastly improved therapy and, consequently, in diminished morbidity and mortality associated with urinary tract problems in the quadriplegic.

HISTORICAL BACKGROUND

Throughout history, numerous wars have resulted in disabling some of the most able-bodied persons in the prime of their lives. The experience gained from the First and Second World War laid the foundation of our present-day management of patients with spinal cord injuries. Not too long ago, the main cause of death after spinal cord injury was renal failure due to urinary tract infection. The most widely used method of treatment was periodic catheterization of distended bladder or suprapubic drainage. In 1917, Thomson-Walker[9] condemned intermittent catheterization. Therefore, Fraser[10] in

1919, used only manual expression of the distended bladder. This resulted in severe hydronephrosis and occasional bladder rupture. When Guttman (1944) revolutionized the management concept by instituting regularly scheduled sterile intermittent catheterization, the high mortality was finally controlled. Lapides (1960) was the first to put forward the interesting concept that sterile catheterization was unnecessary and *clean* intermittent catheterization would suffice. Finally, advances in pharmacotherapy, as well as urinary and penile prosthetics, have altered the quality of survival dramatically.

ACUTE PHASE

This is the phase of "spinal shock," a term coined by Marshall Hall in 1941. Its hallmark is areflexia of the motor and autonomic system below the level of the cervical segment involved. There are no movements of arms or legs, and deep-tendon reflexes are absent. However, there is no decrease in the activity of the external sphincter muscle. The autonomic disturbances consist of loss of sympathetic and parasympathetic activities. Therefore, vasomotor control, bladder, bowel, and sexual functions are at a standstill. In general this phase can persist from eight days to eight weeks.

URODYNAMIC FINDINGS

In spinal shock, bladder filling continues without any sense of distention being perceived by the patient, because there is loss of proprioception. No reflex activity of the bladder muscle is seen, despite overfilling of the bladder. This indicates that the bladder is areflexic. If an electromyographic electrode is inserted into the external urinary sphincter or anal sphincter, normal motor neurons are found to be present. But these sphincters cannot be contracted or relaxed voluntarily by the patient. While the bladder is inactive, the pressure within the membranous urethra is high. The bladder neck is closed as seen on the radiographic study of the bladder.

MANAGEMENT

The aim of management is to relieve urinary retention, to prevent overdistention of the bladder, and to control urinary tract infection. Overdistention of the bladder can cause myogenic failure of the detrussor muscle. This is further aggravated by urinary tract infection. Ultimately the recovery of bladder function is considerably delayed and sometimes seriously impaired.

The initial injury that caused quadriplegia is often associated with other multiple injuries requiring initial intensive care. Diuresis in these patients is a common occurrence; hence, accurate records of intake and output are mandatory. A small (14 F or less) self retaining indwelling catheter is preferred. As soon as the patient's condition is stable the catheter should be removed. It is seldom necessary to retain the catheter beyond 72 hours. This is an average time in which vital signs become stable.

On occasion there may be severe trauma to the penile perineal region as well. This may make insertion of a urethral catheter difficult or even impossible. In these circumstances a narrow-gauge cystostomy tube may be inserted by trochar under local anesthesia. As soon as intermittent catheterization can be instituted, the suprapubic tube should be removed.

During the phase of bladder areflexia due to spinal shock, there is no justification for employing a Crede maneuver. Manual expression of the bladder to express urine simply causes very high pressure within the bladder, resulting in vesico-urethral reflux and hydronephrosis.

A regimen of sterile intermittent catheterization is instituted as soon as the patient's condition allows. The last 40 years have seen a great evolution in the management of quadriplegic patients. Sterile intermittent catheterization was started by Sir Ludwig Guttman in 1949.[2] It remains the management of choice.

A sterile catheter pack is used each time, and strict sterile technique is employed. After dressing in a sterile gown, gloves, and mask, the glans penis is cleansed. Sterile drapes are used. A lubricated plastic catheter, size F10 or the equivalent, is gently introduced into the bladder. Gentle suprapubic pressure is sometime needed to empty the bladder completely. The catheter is removed immediately.

While as a rule catheterization is performed four times a day, this frequency may be varied somewhat depending on urinary output. During the first week after cervical injury there is initial water retention and resultant oliguria. In this phase, twice-daily catheterization may suffice. This is soon followed by a profound diuresis. Appropriately, catheterization more than four times a day may be required to prevent overdistention of the bladder. The fluid intake should be restricted to adjust the catheterized volume to between 400 and 500 ml.

Antibiotics are not used routinely. Initially, urine cultures are performed three times a week. If significant infection is reported on repeated cultures, it is vigorously treated by suitable antibiotics.

This technique of sterile intermittent catheterization has proven itself to be safe and highly efficient over many years of follow-up.

Lapides in 1972[3] modified the concept of sterile intermittent catheterization. He acknowledged the importance of not leaving the catheter indwelling. However, he argued that important factors are not the sterility of the catheter, but removal of residual urine and prevention of ischemia of the bladder mucosa that is caused by overdistention.

The presence of a foreign body in the bladder usually results in urinary tract infection within 48 to 72 hours. It becomes impossible to eradicate this infection permanently unless the foreign body is renewed. Prolonged use of indwelling catheters should therefore be discouraged. The recovery of bladder functions is greatly compromised by this persistent, chronic urinary tract infection. The other complications of indwelling urethral catheter are severe urethritis, penoscrotal fistula (8.8%), vesicovaginal fistula, and bladder stones (49.1%),[4] as well as epididymitis (12.8%), renal stones (13%), and hydronephrosis (11.4%).

Tidal drainage, popularized by Munro,[5] is rarely used today.

The use of suprapubic cystostomy also perpetuates urinary tract infection. In the period after World War I it was well recognized that ascending urinary tract infection was the main threat to the long-term survival of patients. Long-term use of suprapubic catheters reduces the bladder capacity to a considerable degree. This makes subsequent bladder rehabilitation extremely difficult. However, the factors responsible were poorly recognized. After World War II, a large number of spinal cord injury patients were treated with suprapubic cystostomy. At the time, it was widely (but mistakenly) believed that early suprapubic drainage prevented the dreaded urinary tract infection. However, not only do suprapubic catheters have all the disadvantages of indwelling urethral catheters, but, in addition extremely contracted bladders, hydroureter and hydronephrosis are commonly seen after their use. These complications are due to the chronic inflammatory changes of the bladder, ureters, and surrounding tissues. Therefore, the use of suprapubic cystostomy cannot be endorsed at any stage of treatment.

Another method of bladder drainage—cutaneous vesicostomy—enjoyed a period of brief popularity, but it has not proven to be very useful over the long term.

Parasympathomimetic drugs such as bethanechol chloride do not hasten the recovery. In fact, by raising urethral pressure they may actually prove to be harmful.

FOLLOW-UP

Intermittent catheterization (four times in 24 hours) is continued in quadriplegic patients, both male and female, until reflex function of the bladder has fully returned. This may take up to eight weeks.

Urine cultures are performed three times a week in this early phase. If infection free, cultures may be performed on a weekly basis.

Urodynamic tests may be repeated to determine the status of recovery of the bladder.

POSTRECOVERY PHASE

There are no guidelines that help to predict the exact timing of recovery of bladder and urethral function. It may take from eight days to eight weeks. In the postrecovery phase cystometry is the most useful test for assessing the reflex activity of the bladder. However, if detailed knowledge of bladder and urethral function is desired, the following urodynamic tests may be employed to advantage:

1. *Uroflowmetry* for determining the rate of urinary flow.

2. *Cystometry* for assessing the strength of bladder contractile force.

3. *Abdominal pressure measurement* for measuring the effect of straining during micturition.

4. *Electromyography* of the external sphincter for determining contraction or relaxation of the external sphincter striate muscle component.

5. *Urethral pressure* may be measured at the proximal and membranous urethral level.

6. *Fluoroscopic study* of micturition can define the anatomic details of bladder neck and urethra. This study is most meaningful when combined with the above tests.

It is important that all these tests be performed by an individual knowledgeable in the field. Erroneous conclusions may cause irreversible damage to the patient by ill-advised surgery. Based on urodynamic findings, two broad categories of patients can be recognized:

1. *Hyper-reflexic bladder with coordinated sphincter (external and internal).*— As reflex activity of the bladder returns, involuntary bladder contractions are accompanied by a coordinated opening of the bladder neck and relaxation of external sphincter. This results in good periodic emptying of the bladder.

2. *Hyperreflexic bladder with a dyssynergic sphincter (external and/or internal).*—The involuntary bladder contraction is accompanied by an inappropriate closure of the external sphincter. This results in poor emptying residual urine. Classically these patients will manifest the signs and symptoms of autonomic hyperreflexia if the bladder is allowed to distend.

MANAGEMENT OF THE CHRONIC STAGE (POSTRECOVERY PLAN)

The primary goals of treatment are the following:

1. To preserve renal function by control of residual urine, urinary tract infection, and vesico-ureteral reflux.

2. To maintain continence whenever possible.

3. To achieve a catheter free state.

In order to achieve these goals, mechanical, surgical, and pharmacologic methods are employed.

HYPERREFLEXIC BLADDER WITH COORDINATED SPHINCTER

In this group of patients the recovery of reflex contraction of the bladder takes place. The important determinant of eventual outcome is the behavior of sphincter mechanism during this reflex bladder contraction. The internal sphincter (bladder neck) relaxes, as does the external sphincter. Therefore, voiding can take place with satisfactory emptying.

In the early phase of recovery, the bladder contraction may not be strong enough to expel most of the urine. Therefore, intermittent catheterization cannot be discontinued abruptly and prematurely. There are, however, some guidelines that can be used to help in deciding when bladder training can be started.

The oral intake of fluid is adjusted so that the amount of urine produced is approximately 1,500 ml in 24 hours. The patient is encouraged to initiate reflex voiding by recognizing and employing identified "trigger" points. These maneuvers may vary, but generally consist of suprapubic tap, crede, valsalva, or anal stretch. Once the patient learns to trigger voiding, an accurate record of volume voided is maintained. It is immediately followed by catheterization and post-void residual urine is measured. As the residual urine volume decreases the number of catheterizations is reduced. The post-void residual urine should be recorded accurately. When it is less than 150 ml (and only then), intermittent catheterization can be discontinued. Periodic spot checks, however, are necessary. Urine cultures are performed weekly. If infection is detected, it is vigorously treated with appropriate antimicrobial agents as determined by culture and sensitivity tests.

As a preventive measure, in the event of an unexpected bladder evacuation, many male patients will wear a condom catheter attached to a leg bag. On female patients, though, since there are no appliances available to fit the female genitalia as an alternative, bladder contractions may be controlled by using anticholinergic drugs. The commonly used agent is oxybutynin (Ditropan®) at a dose of 5 mg orally three times a day. The dosage may be regulated according to therapeutic response. However, in many patients, these agents are not effective. Excessive use of this drug may paralyze the bladder and cause urinary retention. Sacral nerve block has given good results in selected patients, and may solve this therapeutic dilemma.

HYPERREFLEXIC BLADDER WITH DYSSYNERGIC SPHINCTER (INTERNAL AND/OR EXTERNAL)

In this group of patients the reflex activity of the bladder is accompanied by inappropriate contraction of the internal sphincter (bladder neck) and/or the external sphincter—so-called vesico-urethral dyssynergia. Despite the strong bladder contraction and very high intravesical pressure, bladder emptying is inefficient. The EMG of the external sphincter reveals that its activity inappropriately increases during reflex bladder contraction. Observation of micturition under fluoroscopy fails to reveal adequate opening of the bladder neck despite extremely strong bladder contractions. The measurement of urethral pressure reveals a rise in pressure rather than an expected fall during micturition. This constitutes internal sphincter dyssynergia.

It is imperative that the presence of sphincter dyssynergia be diagnosed properly. Intravesical pressure rises steeply during reflex bladder contraction against a closed sphincter mechanism. High intravesical pressure renders the bladder mucosa ischemic, thereby causing a breakdown in its defense mechanism. This sets the stage for dangerous urinary tract infection. The high intravesical pressure, in addition to causing bladder diverticula, also damages the antireflux mechanism of the ureterovesical junction. This causes reflux of urine from the bladder into the kidneys. Obviously, any infection present in the bladder is carried into the kidneys, and pyelonephritis results. Eventually it causes renal failure.

AUTONOMIC HYPERREFLEXIA

The high intravesical pressure in quadriplegic patients also brings about autonomic hyperreflexia (dysreflexia).[6] Because of the interruption of spinal pathways, the afferent impulses arising from the distended bladder cannot reach the brain. As a result, these afferent impulses are channelled into the thoracic sympathetic nerves, causing profound sympathetic stimulation of the end-organs supplied by them. The profound wide ranging derangements that result are as follows:

1. Constriction of the visceral arterioles supplied by the splanchnic nerves. This intense vasoconstriction causes a sudden severe rise in blood pressure. Throbbing headache is experienced by the patient. Cerebrovascular hemorrhage may result.
2. Since baroreceptors in the carotid arch are intact, bradycardia results. This compensatory mechanism of the baroreceptors is an attempt to lower the seriously elevated blood pressure.
3. Piloerection takes place due to the sympathetic stimulation of hair follicles.
4. Sweat glands, supplied by sympathetic nerves, release their secretions, while vasoconstriction of the skin reduces body surface temperature.
5. The bladder neck (internal sphincter) is supplied by the sympathetic nervous system. Therefore, in the event of sympathetic stimulation, closure of bladder neck takes place (internal sphincter dyssynergia). This causes the in-

travesical pressure to rise further, thereby setting up a vicious cycle. It must be understood that autonomic hyperreflexia can be initiated by distention of an abdominal viscera, particularly rectum.

PHARMACOLOGIC MANAGEMENT

The internal urethral sphincter (bladder neck) is innervated primarily by α-adrenergic sympathetic nerves. Hence, α-adrenergic blocking agents are sometimes useful in counteracting internal sphincter dyssynergia. Experience has shown that they are most effective in partial injuries. In complete injuries, their value is much less certain. Traditionally, phenoxybenzamine, 10 mg three times a day, has been used. Recently it has been shown that this agent is carcinogenic. Therefore, other alpha blockers are being used, e.g., Minipress, 5 mg three times a day, with the dosage to be adjusted according to the therapeutic response.

For the external sphincter (striate muscle component) dyssynergia, sphincterotomy[7] incising the external sphincter muscle endoscopically remains the most effective treatment. On occasion, dantrolene sodium, 25 mg three times a day, may reduce spasticity and improve voiding.

After properly treating the dyssynergia, further efforts are directed toward bladder training with a view toward achieving a "balanced bladder." In specialized centers for spinal cord injury patients, 95% of patients should be able to achieve a catheter-free state.

CAUSES OF UNBALANCED BLADDER FUNCTION

A state of unbalance exists if, after good recovery of reflex bladder contraction, residual urine is still more than 200 ml. If intermittent catheterization is necessary for longer than 20 weeks from the time of injury, a thorough urodynamic evaluation is needed in order to identify the cause of unbalance.

The most important problem to identify is the persistence of detrusor-sphincter dyssynergia causing outflow obstruction. Episodes of autonomic dysreflexia are pathognomic of outflow obstruction and is treated by external sphincterotomy. If sphincterotomy has already been done, it should be revised. Other causes of unbalance, such as prostatic enlargement, bladder neck fibrosis, and myogenic failure due to prolonged distention of bladder, may also be found.

THE ULTIMATE AIM

In the early stages of spinal cord injury, every effort must be made to prevent urinary tract infection and overdistention of the bladder. The isolated spinal cord will regain local reflexes which must then be properly directed by appropriate training. Reflexes that are detrimental to the patient, such as detrusor sphincter dyssynergia, must be recognized early and proper measures taken. The dangers of autonomic hyperreflexia should be fully appreciated. The ultimate aim is full rehabilitation of the patient.

REFERENCES

1. Rossier B.A., Bushra A.F.: From intermittent catheterization to catheter freedom via urodynamics—A tribute to Herr Ludwig Guttman. *Paraplegia* 17:73–85, 1979.
2. Guttman L., Frankel H.: The value of intermittent catheterization in the early management of traumatic paraplegia and Tetraplegia. *Paraplegia* 4:63–84, 1966.
3. Lapides J.: Neurogenic bladder: Principles of treatment. in *Urol. Clin. North Am.,* February 1984, vol. 1, No. 1, pp. 89–90.
4. Jacobson S.A., Bors E.: Spinal cord injury in Vietnamese combat. *Paraplegia* 7:263–281, 1970.
5. Munro D.: Tidal drainage and cystometry in the treatment of sepsis associated with spinal cord injury. *N. Engl. J. Med.* 229:6–14, 1943.
6. Guttman L.: *Spinal cord injury: Comprehensive Management and Research,* ed. 2. Blackwell Scientific Publications, chap. 26.
7. Perkash I.: Problems of decatheterization in long-term spinal cord injury patients. *J. Urol.* 124:249–253, 1980.

8. Perkash I.: Intermittent catheterization failure and approach to bladder rehabilitation in spinal cord injury patients. *Arch. Phys. Med. Rehabil.* 59:9–17, 1978.
9. Thomson-Walker J.W.: The bladder in gunshot and other injuries of the spinal cord. *Lancet* 1:173, 1917.
10. Fraser F.: Urethras and their orifices in gunshot wounds of the spine. *Br. Med. J.* 1:293, 1919.

6

Urinary Tract Infections

Robert A. Press, M.D., Ph.D.

SCOPE OF THE PROBLEM

URINARY TRACT INFECTION is the most frequent infectious cause of morbidity and mortality in the patient with spinal cord injury, and represents the leading cause of fever in this group.[1] Although the bladder is the most common portion of the urinary tract that becomes infected (i.e., cystitis), urethritis, epididymitis, orchitis, periurethral and scrotal abscesses, and pyelonephritis also occur with significant frequency. Urinary calculi may form after repeated infections, and these may in turn become infected; or infection may occur proximal to the resulting obstruction.[2] The most frequent source of septicemia in the spinal cord injury patient is the urinary tract.[3]

Because of spasticity or flaccidity of the bladder, nearly all such patients require indwelling catheterization at some point. The catheter serves as a portal of entry for bacteria, and virtually 100% of patients with indwelling Foley catheters eventually become infected. In most instances, such infection consists of asymptomatic bacteriuria (see below), but sometimes infection is symptomatic. In this regard, it must be remembered that most patients with spinal cord injury will lack the normal sensations associated with urinary tract infections (e.g., dysuria, urgency, back pain, etc.) and the only "symptom" may be fever, with elevation of white blood cell (WBC) count sometimes present as an additional sign.

INDWELLING FOLEY VERSUS INTERMITTENT CATHETERIZATION

Most patients with spinal cord injury require at least some period of catheterization. A single catheterization is associated with a 1% to 3% risk of infection, with bacteria introduced in this instance from the periurethral area. Once the catheter is inserted, bacteria may enter the bladder via the interface between the catheter and the urethral meatus. However, more commonly, contamination occurs either at the point of connection of the collecting tube and the catheter, or in the collection bag or urimeter, with retrograde flow to the bladder.[4]

Essentially 100% of patients with indwelling catheters will become infected. Such infections usually consist of asymptomatic bacteriuria (defined as more than 100,000 bacteria per milliliter without symptoms), with symptomatic infection generally occurring only when the catheter becomes obstructed or, through manipulation, traumatizes the mucosa. Regarding the latter, it should be noted that such obstruction or trauma can lead to infection of contiguous areas, e.g., epididymitis or periurethral abscess.

Not only do spinal cord injury patients with indwelling catheters develop bacteriuria, but in one study about 12% developed renal calculi within the first three years of injury, and 18% developed reflux in long-term follow-ups.[5] As noted previously, each urethral catheterization is associated with a 1% to 3% incidence of infection, and the trauma of catheterization itself may lead to bacteremia, especially if the patient's bladder is already colonized by bacteria. Therefore, in most patients with poor bladder function and high residual volumes of urine, indwelling Foley catheterization and suprapubic cystostomy have been used for bladder drainage. The management differs for the spinal cord injury patient. This is mainly because many if not most of these patients are young, and therefore catheterization can be performed with relatively little trauma.

It has been found in many studies that intermittent catheterization, performed aseptically by a "nontouch" technique every six to eight hours, is preferable to an indwelling Foley in these patients.[6] The nontouch technique is an aseptic method of self-catheterization. The catheter is manipulated while wrapped in sterile gauze. Gloves are not used, but the patient's hands are never in contact with the catheter. Disposable catheter systems are also available enclosed within sterile sleeves; these systems are of course more expensive than the others, since they can only be used once and then discarded. The method has advantages from the standpoint of bladder training, infection, and the complications of infection.

Regarding bladder training, the nontouch technique has been used to allow detrusor muscle automaticity to evolve. It has been found that such patients generally develop fewer urinary tract infections than do those with indwelling Foley catheters, and those infections that do develop are generally caused by more sensitive organisms.[3] The latter phenomenon is probably secondary to the fact that patients with indwelling Foley catheters have usually been the recipients of multiple course of antibiotics for their urinary tract infections, and that some of these courses of antibiotics may have been unnecessary. (See section on "treatment" below.) Regarding the complications of infection, the incidence of hydronephrosis was decreased to 7.4%, ureteral reflux to 4.4%, and renal calculi to 1.7%.[6] Urethral fistulae and diverticula from periurethral abscesses were also markedly decreased in incidence in patients who were catheterized intermittently.

CARE OF INDWELLING FOLEY CATHETER

Despite the advantage of intermittent catheterization for most young patients with spinal cord injury, some spinal-cord-injured patients, especially older ones, are unable to tolerate this method of bladder drainage. This may be due to the trauma of catheterization in this population, or to the presence of incontinence with resultant contamination of decubitus ulcers. For these patients, indwelling Foley catheters are preferable.

Proper catheter care may delay the onset of bacteriuria and prevent bacteremia.[7] Catheters should be inserted aseptically. Following insertion, they must be properly secured to prevent movement, which leads to urethral trauma and introduction of bacteria. Catheterized patients should have once- or twice-daily perineal care, including cleansing of the meatal-catheter junction with an antiseptic soap to prevent the introduction of bacteria at this location.

A sterile closed drainage system should always be used. Continuous irrigation with antibiotic solution (e.g., neomycin-polymyxin) or acetic acid has not been shown to be more effective in delaying the onset of infection than the closed drainage system.

The catheter and the collection tube should not be disconnected unless irrigation of an obstructed catheter is required. When this is done, aseptic techniques should be employed. If frequent irrigations are necessary to ensure patency, a three-way Foley catheter with continuous irrigation should be used. Each time the catheter is disconnected, bacteria may be introduced into the system. Nonobstructed downhill flow should be maintained at all times. This requires maintenance of collecting bags below the level of the bladder. Otherwise, bacteria in a contaminated collecting bag can be introduced into the bladder more easily by retrograde flow. The collecting bag should be emptied frequently, and poorly functioning or obstructed catheters should be replaced. If bags are inverted or raised above the level of the patient's bladder, the tubing should be clamped. Urine for chemical determinations should be sterilely obtained from the drainage bag.

Catheters should routinely be changed only when obstruction or contamination occurs, or when concretions can be palpated in the catheter. Changing catheters every few days or weeks only serves to introduce new bacteria or to traumatize the urinary tract, thereby increasing the chance for bacteremia to occur.

Some experts feel that a silicone catheter should be used in cases where the catheter is to be in place for longer than five days, since this material may be less subject to bacterial colonization than latex, which is usually used in the manufacture of catheters. In addition, the use of methenamine plus acidification may control bacterial growth, and acidification may retard stone formation. Good urine flow should be maintained to prevent obstruction, so daily fluid intake of at least 2,000 ml is generally recommended.

URINE CULTURES IN CATHETERIZED PATIENTS

A urine culture should routinely be obtained at the time the patient is catheterized. It should also be done periodically while the catheter is in place (e.g., every few weeks), and just before the removal of the catheter.

Urine for culture from catheterized patients should be aspirated from the distal part of the catheter using a small-gauge needle and sterile syringe. The catheter should first be prepared with tincture of iodine or betadine. It must be noted that quantitative culture of urine so obtained may not accurately reflect the quantitative culture of bladder urine. There is evidence that the inner surface of the catheter becomes colonized by bacteria accounting for this disparity.

TREATMENT OF INFECTION IN CATHETERIZED PATIENTS

The bacteriuria that inevitably occurs in the catheterized patient should not routinely be treated with the catheter in place, since this leads to colonization with more resistant organisms.

Patients can become septic from this source, but this usually occurs only if the catheter becomes obstructed, is manipulated, or is irrigated. In these instances, patients should be treated with appropriate antibiotics based on culture results. It may also be advisable to treat asymptomatic bacteriuria in diabetic patients, since such individuals do often go on to symptomatic infection. Similarly, it may be wise to treat patients with asymptomatic *Proteus* infections if they are known stone-formers, since infection with this urea-splitting organism will predispose the patient to stone formation.

To sterilize the urine, the catheter must be changed during the therapy, since it will be impossible to eradicate all the bacteria from the tip, which will serve as a nidus with consequent reinfection of the urine after the antibiotic therapy is stopped.

It must be emphasized that, if fever develops in a patient with an indwelling Foley catheter, the physician should look assiduously for another source of infection before ascribing it to the urinary tract. Under any circumstances treatment should include antibiotics that will appropriately cover urinary tract organisms as well as other possible sources of infection.

Asymptomatic bacteriuria should be treated prior to any urinary tract instrumentation, e.g., cystoscopy, since this procedure might lead to bacteremia. Such antibiotic coverage should probably begin the night before such manipulation.

Finally, some experts suggest that asymptomatic bacteriuria should be treated if the catheter is to be removed, with removal performed within 48 hours of beginning an appropriate antibiotic regimen.[8]

TREATMENT OF INFECTION IN PATIENTS UNDERGOING INTERMITTENT CATHETERIZATION

In contrast to the situation with an indwelling Foley catheter, urinary tract infection in patients undergoing intermittent catheterization should always be treated, even if the infection is totally asymptomatic. The reason for this is twofold. First, these patients may develop substantial residual volumes of urine in the bladder at times. If the bladder wall is stretched and the urine contained therein is infected, bacteremia may ensue. Second, if the urine is infected, bacteremia may also occur during the catheterization itself, should there be any associated trauma to the mucosa.

In general, no prophylactic antibiotics are recommended for

this group of patients. Urine should be cultured periodically, with each infection treated with an appropriate antibiotic.

ETIOLOGY OF URINARY TRACT INFECTIONS IN SPINAL CORD INJURY PATIENTS

In the general population, hospital-acquired *Escherichia coli* is by far the most common cause of urinary tract infection. In the spinal-cord-injured patient who undergoes intermittent catheterization, this organism also predominates.[3] However, this is not the case in spinal-cord-injured patients with neurogenic bladders with persistently large residual volumes of urine, or in patients with indwelling Foley catheters. Large residual volumes, with resultant stasis, are responsible for the growth of microorganisms, since urine is a relatively good culture medium. As outlined previously, patients with indwelling Foley catheters virtually all become infected. In these populations, *Pseudomonas aeruginosa, Klebsiella* species, and *Proteus mirabilis* predominate as causes of urinary tract infections. These organisms are likely present secondary to multiple previous courses of antibiotic therapy, with consequent selection of resistance.

Of the gram-positive organisms that occur, *Enterococcus* predominates, with *Staphylococcus saprophyticus, Staphylococcus epidermidis,* and *Staphylococcus aureus* occurring to a lesser degree. Infection with *S. aureus* should prompt a search for an additional focus of infection, since this species usually arrives in the urinary tract via a hematogenous route. Alternatively, its presence may indicate an abscess in the prostate or the periurethral area.

Candida cystitis does not usually reflect systemic candidiasis. Rather, it commonly follows catheterization in a patient receiving broad spectrum antibiotic therapy.

A Gram's stain of the urine is helpful in defining the etiologic agent, and should certainly be done if the patient is septic or if no recent urine culture is available, unless broad-spectrum antibiotic coverage is to be used empirically. One organism per oil immersion field of unspun urine roughly correlates with 100,000 organisms per cubic centimeter. The presence of white blood cell casts indicates upper urinary tract involvement.

Although microscopic examination is a rapid diagnostic tool, quantitative culture of the urine is necessary for definitive diagnosis. More than 100,000 organisms per cubic centimeter of urine obtained by clean catch or catheterization is considered to represent significant bacteriuria. It should be remembered that the figure of 100,000 organisms per cubic centimeter was determined for gram-negative rods. No one really knows the significant number of gram-positive organisms, although 100,000 has been adopted by convention. Dilute urine secondary to forcing of fluids may lead to a misleadingly low colony count. Any number of organisms found in urine obtained by suprapubic aspiration of the bladder is considered significant.

The urine must not be permitted to stand at room temperature before culture, since this allows organisms to multiply. Rather, it should be refrigerated if it cannot be cultured within an hour after it is obtained.

The pH of the urine in a patient with positive findings on microscopic examination should give a clue to the cause of the infection. A pH of 8.0 or above may indicate a *Proteus* infection, since this organism splits urea, leading to NH_3 production and alkalinization. However, vegetarians and persons who take sodium bicarbonate to prevent uric acid stone formation may also have alkaline urine.

CHOICE OF AN ANTIBIOTIC AGENT

When an infection requires treatment, therapy should be guided by in vitro sensitivity data whenever possible. Such data should generally be available since, as outlined earlier, routine cultures should be obtained from patients with indwelling Foley catheters or those undergoing intermittent catheterization. The least toxic, narrowest spectrum, least expensive agent should be used whenever possible.

Sulfa drugs are a good choice for the treatment of cystitis caused by susceptible gram-negative rods, especially since they are quite inexpensive. For sulfisoxazole, the adult dosage is 500 mg to 1 gm four times a day. For sulfamethoxazole, the dose is 1 gm twice a day. The standard length of treatment for cystitis in the spinal cord injury patient is seven to ten days.

Another first-line drug for cystitis caused by susceptible organisms is tetracycline or its derivatives in a dose of 250 mg four times daily. The drug should not be used in children, since it causes staining of the teeth. Furthermore, its absorption is decreased by milk or milk products. It is ineffective at pH 8 and therefore will not be efficacious against urea-splitters like *Proteus.*

Low-dose ampicillin in the dose of 250 mg four times daily is also an effective and relatively inexpensive agent. Cephalosporins, like cephalexin (250 mg four times daily), cephradine (250 mg four times daily), and cefadroxil (500 mg twice daily) are also effective, but are more expensive. Nitrofurantoin (100 mg four times daily) and nalidixic acid (1 gm four times daily) are useful, although the former often leads to nausea and vomiting, and the latter is associated with the rapid emergence of resistance.

The combination of trimethoprim (80 mg) and sulfamethoxazole (400 mg) should not be used if the causative organism is sensitive to any of the less expensive, narrower spectrum agents above. However, if the organism is resistant to the above agents, this combination may prove extremely efficacious. The dosage is two tablets twice daily. It should be noted that sulfa-trimethoprim is the agent of choice in patients with a chronic prostatic focus of infection, since trimethoprim is the antimicrobial with optimal penetration of the prostate.

If the patient suffers from an enterococcal cystitis, the drug of choice is ampicillin (250 mg four times daily) or amoxicillin (250 mg three times daily). If an allergy to penicillin exists, erythromycin (500 mg four times daily) may be substituted, but the urine must be alkalinized for this drug to be effective.

The efficacy of therapy may be accurately assessed after 24 to 48 hours, even if in vitro sensitivity data are unavailable. After this time period of appropriate antibiotic therapy, the urine should be sterile, and Gram's stain should confirm this. If organisms are still present in the unspun urine, they are likely to be resistant to the current antibiotic, unless there is some element of obstruction present. Not infrequently, the urine may be sterilized by an antibiotic to which the organism is resistant in vitro. Many of the agents mentioned achieve a concentration in the urine that exceeds that in the standard disc used for testing. At the higher concentration, the bacteria may be sensitive to the agent. If the urine is sterile, there is no need to switch to another antibiotic based on the in vitro data. It must be reemphasized that if the patient has an indwelling Foley catheter, this must be changed at some point during the course of therapy or the patient will relapse after the antimicrobial treatment is discontinued.

When no culture data are available at the time that therapy needs to be begun, empiric therapy should be initiated after a culture is obtained. If a Gram's stain shows the offending organism to be a gram-negative rod, an aminoglycoside with anti-*Pseudomonas* activity (e.g., gentamicin, tobramycin, or amikacin) intramuscularly or intravenously should probably be used pending sensitivity data. The dosage of gentamicin or tobramycin is approximately 1 mg/kg q (8 hours × serum creatinine), while that of amikacin is 7.5 mg/kg q (9 hours × serum creatinine, but not more frequently than q12h). Serum aminoglycoside peak and trough levels should be monitored, but peak levels need not be in the high therapeutic range, since these agents are concentrated in the urine. An alternative to therapy with an aminoglycoside is that with a "third-generation" cephalosporin such as cefoperazone, moxalactam, cefotaxime, ceftazidime, or ceftizoxime, or with imipenem. If the patient is not very sick, and an oral agent is desired, sulfa-trimethoprim (two tablets of single strength twice daily) can be used, but this will not cover *Pseudomonas*.

If no prior culture is available and urine shows gram-positive cocci on Gram's stain, the organism is most likely to be *Enterococcus*, with *Staphylococcus* a less likely possibility. Full coverage would include ampicillin or amoxicillin for the former, and vancomycin (IV) for the latter.

If *Candida* cystitis needs to be treated, continuous bladder irrigation with low-dose amphotericin B (50 mg in 1,000 cc 5% dextrose in water by continuous drip over 24 hours for five days) can be utilized. There is virtually no systemic absorption of the amphotericin through the bladder wall. If the patient is not catheterized, an alternative is 5-fluorocytosine, 50 mg/kg/day (if the patient has normal renal and hepatic function).

If upper urinary tract disease is suspected (e.g., if white blood cell casts are seen in the urine) and especially if the patient is septic, parenteral antibiotic therapy is preferable initially, and is essential if the patient has associated nausea and vomiting. Gram-negative pyelonephritis should initially be treated with one of the broad-spectrum antibiotics discussed previously (aminoglycoside or "third-generation" cephalosporin) pending sensitivities. If gram-positive organisms are seen in the infected urine, the patient should probably be treated initially with vancomycin (500 mg IV every six hours if renal function is normal) pending identification and sensitivities of the organism.

Once sensitivities are known, antibiotic therapy should be adjusted to the least toxic, narrowest spectrum agent.

As with cystitis, within 24 to 48 hours of the institution of appropriate therapy, the urine should be sterile. If this is not the case, obstruction should be suspected and investigated, for example, with an IV pyelogram or ultrasound. Fever and pyuria may persist much longer than bacteriuria in uncomplicated pyelonephritis, and complete defervescence may take up to a week to occur. The usual course of treatment is two weeks, although relapses may occur and require several months of therapy. The proportion of this therapy that needs to be parenteral has not been determined, even when blood cultures are positive. Certainly, uncomplicated pyelonephritis has been successfully treated with oral therapy alone. Many would use slightly higher doses than for simple cystitis (e.g., 2 gm daily of ampicillin instead of 1 gm). As for *Pseudomonas aeruginosa* cystitis, carbenicillin or ticarcillin may be used without an aminoglycoside in pyelonephritis caused by susceptible strains.

COMPLICATIONS AND SEQUELAE OF URINARY TRACT INFECTIONS IN SPINAL CORD INJURY PATIENTS

The urinary tract is the most common source of gram-negative sepsis in spinal cord injury patients. As in gram-negative sepsis of other origins, this may occasionally lead to renal shutdown. This is usually secondary to acute tubular necrosis rather than to overwhelming infection of the kidneys, and most often is reversible. Renal damage as a direct result of the kidney infection (i.e., not secondary to sepsis) is most often quite focal, and although cortical scars may occur in severe cases, little if any lasting decline in renal function is noted. Occasionally, severe pyelonephritis may lead to anuria on the basis of bilateral papillary necrosis or acute cortical necrosis. There are only rare cases of chronic renal failure that can be traced to one or more episodes of acute pyelonephritis.

Occasionally, kidney infection may extend beyond the cortex and renal capsule, to the perinephric fat. In this case a perinephric abscess results.

Infection may predispose to stone formation, especially if *Proteus* is the pathogen. These stones may in turn obstruct the urinary tract, predisposing to repeated episodes of infection. In addition, the stone itself may become the nidus for continuing infection. In either case, cure of the infection usually requires removal of the calculus. Sometimes the infection can be suppressed with long-term antibiotic therapy.

Finally, it must be remembered that infection of any portion of the urinary tract may extend to any other portion, especially with a (potentially) obstructed catheter in place. For example, infection of the bladder may extend to the prostate, epididymis, testicle, or kidney.

REFERENCES

1. Sugarman B., Brown D., Musher D.: Fever and infection in spinal cord injury patients. *J.A.M.A.* 248:66, 1982.
2. Khella L., Stoner E.K.: 101 cases of spinal cord injury. *Am. J. Phys. Med.* 56:21, 1977.
3. Allen J.R.: Infectious complications in patients with spinal cord injury. *J.A.M.A.* 248:83, 1982.
4. Kunin C.M.: *Detection, Prevention and Management of Urinary Tract Infections,* ed. 3. Philadelphia, Lea & Febiger, 1979.
5. Stamey T.A.: *Urinary Infections.* Baltimore, Williams & Wilkins Co., 1972, pp. 250–251.
6. Guttman L., Frankel H.: The value of intermittent catheterization in the early management of traumatic paraplegia and tetraplegia. *Paraplegia* 4:63, 1966.

7. Press R.A.: Urinary tract infections, in Berger S.A. (ed.): *Clinical Manual of Infectious Diseases.* Menlo Park, Calif., Addison-Wesley Co., 1982, pp. 97–111.
8. Kunin C.M.: Indwelling urinary catheter. *J.A.M.A.* 237:1859, 1977.
9. Govan D.E., Butler E.D., Engelsgjerd G.L.: Pathogenesis of urinary tract infections in patients with neurogenic bladder dysfunction. *Urol. Dig.* 7:16, 1968.

7

Sexual Function in Quadriplegia

Arnold Melman, M.D.

MEN AND WOMEN who are quadriplegic are sexual beings!

Only in the last two decades has the significance of this simple statement received appropriate attention. There has been only gradual understanding of the sexual needs of spinal-cord-injured patients, and awareness that these are a significant part of the sum of care needed for rehabilitation. With that realization, multidimensional centers capable of delivering services oriented to the sexual aspects of people with spinal cord injury have been created.

The extent of treatment and type of rehabilitation necessary for the newly quadriplegic person is an individual matter dependent upon the patient's history and type of injury. It is significant whether or not the patient is a man or woman, single or married, with family or alone, adolescent or adult, as well as whether the individual lives in a metropolitan or rural area. The extent of recovery of sexual function will vary according to the level of the spinal lesions and whether or not the cord was completely severed.

SEXUAL POTENTIAL FOR THE QUADRIPLEGIC MALE

Any plan for further therapy and possible function must be considered in the light components of the male sexual response: libido, erection, orgasm, ejaculation, and, in addition, fertility.

LIBIDO

The desire to be sexual is complex and interrelated with the state of physical and psychological health. In a study of 25 men with quadriplegia six months to 21 years after injury (mean, 8.6 years) Phelps et al.[2] reported that patients' feelings of sexual desire did not change as much as their feelings of adequacy or satisfaction. Only 20% of the group reported their desire to be "weak or very weak." In response to the suggestion that plasma sex hormone levels might be altered after spinal cord injury, the same authors measured plasma testosterone in quadriplegic patients and found a normal concentration of hormone.

ERECTION

Ninety percent of men with lesions of the cervical spinal cord are able to experience reflex erections that return from three weeks to six months after injury.[3] Most patients are not able to have psychic erections (i.e., erections generated by sexual thoughts or sights). Therefore, the erections that occur do so as a result of reflex stimulation of the genital area and may last for seconds to many minutes. In one study of 23 men with complete cervical cord lesions, 21 reported reflex erections.[3, 4] Spontaneous erections occurred in 20 of these patients, and 13 patients had attempted intercourse, six successfully. None of these patients experienced orgasm or ejaculation. In 26 men with incomplete cervical cord lesions, seven had psychic erections and 23 had reflex and spontaneous erections. Seventeen patients had successful intercourse.

Comarr[3] has emphasized that "they (the neurologic deficits) do not necessarily permit to base an accurate prognosis of baseline sexual function upon the level and extent of injury in the individual case." Thus, each patient's recovery and sexual capabilities are unique. This concept must be carefully explained by the rehabilitation professional so that the patient is motivated to maximize his sexual capabilities.

ORGASM

Orgasm is the pleasurable sensation derived from the contraction of the skeletal muscle of the pelvic floor. Cole reports (without experimental evidence) that sensation can be derived if the autonomic innervation of the smooth muscle of the pelvic region is intact. Comarr[3] states that none of the patients with complete cervical cord lesions experience orgasm.

EJACULATION AND FERTILITY

Only 1% of quadriplegic patients have been reported to retain spontaneous ejaculatory ability.[3] At present, the artificial induction of ejaculation by electrical stimulation is in the investigatory stage at the Spinal Cord Injury Service in Palo Alto, Calif.[5] That group has developed a rectal probe stimulator capable of causing seminal emission in paraplegic men. In their studies, retrograde ejaculation occurred in five of 12 patients. Neurologic injury to the bladder neck allows the semen to travel from the ejaculatory ducts into the bladder rather than to the outside. However, appropriate collection techniques might be instituted to allow collection of potentially fertile sperm. Nevertheless, there is little information related to sperm production and possible fertility in quadriplegic patients as a result of insufficient testing.

SEXUALITY IN FEMALE QUADRIPLEGIC PATIENTS

Sexual excitement and orgasm can be achieved despite the possible absence of labial and clitorial sensation if appropriate stimulation to the remaining erogenous zones such as lips, ears, neck, and nipples is applied. Bregman,[6] who summarized the results of her own investigation of sexual function in spinal-cord-injured women, concluded that the "psychological role is more important that the physical one."

Quadriplegic women should be capable of normal ovulation, fertility, pregnancy, and delivery. A potential problem during labor is that of rapid elevation of blood pressure because of the phenomenon of autonomic dysreflexia. This complication should be anticipated and dealt with by the obstetrician. (Also see section on autonomic dysreflexia, p. 69.)

Birth control may be a problem in the quadriplegic women because certain devices such as foam and jellies require a manual dexterity for use that usually is not possible in the quadriplegic. Sterilization of the patient's partner or use of condoms may be satisfactory alternatives.

Vaginal lubrication apparently is not a problem for quadriplegic patients, but if deficient it is easily substituted with water-soluble jelly placed on the penis.

SPECIAL CONSIDERATIONS FOR BOTH MEN AND WOMEN

Problems that affect the patient of either sex include unwanted spasticity, as well as bowel and bladder control during sex. For those with severe spastic response, medication (e.g., diazepam) can be taken to relax skeletal muscle. A program of bowel and bladder emptying prior to coitus by the patient with the help of the partner should be treated in an open, frank manner if a problem is anticipated or has occurred.

SEXUAL REHABILITATION

The treating physician is in the unique position of initiating sexual rehabilitation therapy. A discussion of possible sexual function as part of the overall rehabilitative process will help to reduce the anxiety and concern in the patient.

In an earlier report conducted with quadriplegic men, Hetrick[9] noted that 65% of the men discussed sex with some other person, but only 16% had discussions with their physicians about sexual function. Several authors[2, 6] have reported that patients' overall satisfaction with their lives postinjury directly correlated with the degree of sexual activity. Sexual counseling of the patient can be accomplished ideally in specialized centers, and a seminar format may be used for individuals or for families.

Table 7–1 lists a number of centers that specialize in sexual rehabilitation of spinal-cord-injured persons.

Continuing information for patients can be obtained from the following sources:

Accent on Living
P.O. Box 726
Gillum Road and Hyde Drive
Bloomington, IL   61701

Rehabilitation Gazette
4502 Maryland Avenue
St. Louis, MO   63108

Journal of Sexuality and Disability
Human Sciences Press
72 Fifth Avenue
New York, NY   10011

A list of films related to spinal-cord-injured persons is available for purchase or rental from the Multi Media Resource Center, 1525 Franklin Street, San Francisco, CA 94109.

OPTIONS FOR MEN

After the rehabilitative process is complete, the patient may be satisfied with the final degree of sexual performance. If coitus is desired and erection is of sufficient rigidity and duration to allow penetration to the partner's satisfaction, the aim of sexual rehabilitation will have been met. However, if the patient's reflex erection is insufficient, a penile silicone implant may be considered. Two specific types of implants are avail-

TABLE 7–1.—REHABILITATION CENTERS

Craig Hospital
Rocky Mountain Regional Spinal Injury Center
3425 South Clarkson
Englewood, CO 80010   Tel. (303) 761–3040

Institute of Rehabilitation Medicine
Spinal Cord Injury Center
400 East 34 Street
New York, NY 10016   Tel. (212) 340–6105

Moss Rehabilitation Hospital
12th and Tabor Road
Philadelphia, PA 19141   Tel. (215) 329–5715

Rancho Los Amigos Hospital
Spinal Injury Service
7601 East Imperial Highway
Downey, CA 90242   Tel. (213) 922–7605

The Rehabilitation Institute of Chicago
345 East Superior Street
Chicago, IL 60611   Tel. (312) 649–6179

Santa Clara Valley Medical Center
751 South Bascom
Santa Clara, CA 95128   Tel. (408) 279–5116

The Texas Institute for Rehabilitation & Research
P.O. Box 20095
Houston, TX 77025   Tel. (713) 797–1440

VA Hospital, Bronx*
Spinal Cord Injury Service
Veterans Administration Hospital
130 West Kingsbridge Road
Bronx, NY 10468   Tel. (212) 584–9000, ext. 591

VA Hospital, Cleveland*
Spinal Cord Injury Service
Veterans Administration Hospital
10701 East Boulevard
Cleveland, OH 44106   Tel. (216) 791–3800

VA Hospital, West Roxbury*
Spinal Cord Injury Service
Veterans Administration Hospital
1400 VFW Parkway
West Roxbury, MA 02132   Tel. (617) 323–7700, ext. 210

    *For veterans only.

able. The first is a semirigid device that maintains constant length and diameter of the penis that will allow vaginal penetration at any time without the need of help by the partner to initiate tumescence. The other is an inflatable device; the penis is flaccid until a pumping mechanism in the scrotum is activated. The disadvantage is that active intervention by the partner is necessary for intercourse. The principal complication that may occur in paraplegic and quadriplegic men with permanently implanted penile prosthetic devices is erosion of the device either through the skin or, more frequently, into the urethra. The generalized atrophy that occurs after spinal cord injury causes a thinning of the tunica albuginea, which is the tough fibroelastic covering of the corpus cavernosum. Thus, the constant pressure of the silicone device may result in eventual erosion. Accurate data are not available for the actual incidence of this occurrence, but a rate of 25% with either device is probable.

REFERENCES

1. Cole T.M.: Sexuality and physical disabilities. *Arch. Sex. Behav.* 4:389–403, 1975.
2. Phelps G., Brown M., Chen J., et al.: Sexual experience and plasma testosterone levels in male veterans after spinal cord injury. *Arch. Phys. Med. Rehabil.* 64:47–52, 1983.
3. Comarr A.E.: Sexual function among patients with spinal cord injury. *Urol. Int.* 25:134–168, 1970.
4. Comarr A.E.: Sex classification and expectations among quadriplegics and paraplegics. *Sexuality and Disability* 1:252–259, 1978.
5. Martin D.E., Warner H., Crenshaw T.L., et al.: Initiation of erection and semen release by rectal probe electrostimulation (RPE). *J. Urol.* 129–642, 1983.
6. Bregman S.: Sexuality and social rehabilitation in women after spinal cord injury, in Ami Sha'ked (ed.): *Human Sexuality and Rehabilitation Medicine; Sexual Functioning Following Spinal Cord Injury.* Baltimore, Williams & Wilkins Co., 1981.
7. Bruyere S.: Sexual aspects of spinal cord injury: The state of the art, in Ami Sha'ked (ed.): *Human Sexuality and Rehabilitation Medicine; Sexual Functioning Following Spinal Cord Injury.* Baltimore, Williams & Wilkins Co., 1981.

8. Cole T.M.: Sexual problems of paraplegic women. *Medical Aspects of Human Sexuality* 19:105, 1976.
9. Hetrick W.R.: Sexuality following functional transsection of the spinal cord. *Dissert. Abst.* 288:5206, 1968.
10. Chipouras S.: Ten sexuality programs for spinal cord injured persons. *Sexuality and Disability* 2:301–321, 1979.

8

Gastrointestinal Complications

THE GASTROINTESTINAL COMPLICATIONS of quadriplegia appear both in the acute and chronic state. The unusual presentation of usual gastrointestinal disturbances must be perceived by the physician so that grave errors in clinical judgment can be avoided in these patients.

INNERVATION OF BOWEL

The neurogenic bowel can only be understood in the light of normal gastrointestinal tract physiology. Since normal innervation of bowel depends on nerve input from the multiple spinal levels, the site of the injury will have a major bearing on the degree and kind of dysfunction produced. In view of the fact that neurologic function of the bowel depends on interaction at several levels between the components of the autonomic and voluntary nervous systems, the degree of impairment is not always predictable. This interaction is responsible for the frequently unexpected constellations of symptoms occurring in spinal cord injury patients.

Normal function of the bowel depends on the following: (1) parasympathetic control: the vagus nerve supplies the parasympathetic innervation of the esophagus, stomach, small intestine, and ascending and transverse colons. It is responsible for increased peristalsis and secretions. The pudendal nerve, in turn, fulfills the same function for the descending colon and rectosigmoid. (2) Sympathetic control of the gut arises from T-4 to L-3. Synapses take place at the celiac ganglion and mesenteric plexus. Sympathetic innervation has the effect of diminishing peristalsis and secretions. (3) The only area in the GI tract under voluntary control is the external anal sphincter. Cortical input is inhibitory, thus allowing voluntary control of defecation. The musculature of the pelvic floor and abdominal wall (also under voluntary control) is normally responsible for facilitating (or inhibiting) expulsion of bowel contents. In this sense, at least, these muscles and those of the external anal sphincter must be thought of as a functioning unit.

The vagus, which is a cranial nerve, is spared in spinal cord injury. In high spinal cord injury, there is interruption of the sympathetic pathway. Thus, in cervical spinal cord injury, there is usually disruption of sympathetic control of the entire transverse colon and rectum. In contrast to this is the maintenance of vagal or parasympathetic innervation to the level of the beginning of the descending large bowel. Below this point there is a loss of parasympathetic control because of interruption, by the injury, of S-2, 3, 4 which join into the pudendal nerve. Thus, there is a disproportion between the normal motility of the areas above the upper descending colon and the diminished motility in the remaining colon and rectosigmoid. The external anal sphincter is therefore deprived of cortical (voluntary) control, and the rectum can only empty reflexly.

CLINICAL ASPECTS

The physician's interpretation of location, severity, periodicity, and quality of pain is an essential part of the evaluation of the non–spinal-cord-injured patient with abdominal complaints. However, in dealing with the spinal cord injury patient, the physician cannot expect the above criteria to be helpful in the same way. Both spontaneous pain, as well as tenderness, may be muted, referred, or even completely absent, so that one has to depend on other findings. These include (1) spasticity of the abdominal wall, (2) abdominal distention, (3) vomiting, and (4) fever.

It can reasonably be said, therefore, that systemic complaints in a sense "take over" for localized symptoms and findings, and have to be carefully evaluated when they arise. It must also be emphasized that quadriplegics frequently look relatively "well" even during acute or even catastrophic gastrointestinal episodes.

SPECIFIC SYMPTOMS AND FINDINGS

PAIN

Due to the disruption of visceral sensory fibers in spinal cord injury, visceral pain is perceived vaguely or in a referred fashion. The most common localization of referred pain is from the abdomen to the shoulder blade, flank, inguinal area, and umbilicus. The quality of the referred pain is usually dull and rarely lancinating. It is sensed as more of a discomfort than a pain, and is usually associated with a generally "upset" feeling.

ABDOMINAL SPASTICITY

Rigidity and guarding of the abdominal wall are not usually seen in quadriplegics. On the other hand, abdominal wall spasticity in the quadriplegic with an acute abdomen is quite common.

ABDOMINAL DISTENTION AND ILEUS

Although ileus is expected in the period of spinal shock immediately after injury, it is unusual for bowel sounds to remain absent for more than 48 hours. Active peristalsis almost always begins after the first week.

After the above time has elapsed, absent bowel sounds in the quadriplegic has the same significance as in any other patient. This finding, together with abdominal distention, speaks for an acute abdomen in these patients. Abdominal distention must be interpreted carefully, however. Because of the weakened musculature the abdomen of the quadriplegic appears enlarged, and therefore distention can only be diagnosed as an increase in abdominal size as compared to "baseline."

FEVER AND AUTONOMIC CRISIS

Fever is as always an excellent indicator in the diagnosis of acute gastrointestinal problems of quadriplegics. However, in these patients, rectal temperature rarely goes above 101°F, whereas in urosepsis a much higher fever is usually seen.[6] Autonomic crisis may be another sign of acute abdomen in a spinal-cord-injured patient. For a complete description of this entity see the cardiovascular chapter.

SPECIFIC ENTITIES

EARLY AND LATE ILEUS

In acute spinal cord injury, adynamic ileus is the rule. Although we know that it is "normal" for spinal-cord-injured patients in the immediate postinjury phase to have paralytic ileus, the burden of proof is on the physician in diagnosing associated abdominal trauma. Diagnostic peritoneal lavage is very helpful and should be done as soon as possible after injury. This procedure has a high (more than 90%) success rate for the diagnosis of intra-abdominal hemorrhage.[1]

Sepsis and pulmonary complications are known to be responsible for undue prolongation of the period of early ileus and should be looked for in these instances.

Even if there has been normal resumption of peristalsis approximately one week after injury, ileus may occur months after the injury. Anorexia, distention, nausea, vomiting, and absence of bowel sounds are the keys to diagnosis. Deflation of the gut with nasogastric suction and intravenous fluids usually reverses this condition promptly. However, this condition must be differentiated from potentially more ominous intraperitoneal episodes (to be discussed below). Absence of fever and of shoulder tip pain and absence of significant leukocytosis all speak against intra-abdominal catastrophe, and for the benign conditions described above.

GASTROPARESIS

This condition which is usually only seen in non–spinal-cord-injured patients in diabetes mellitus, hypothyroidism, and hypocalcemia, as well as in abdominal trauma, is frequently seen in quadriplegia in association with ileus. Meclopropamide and neostigmine have been used for the relief of gastroparesis with good results.[3]

STRESS ULCER

Increased gastrin production has been described as a sequela of CNS injury. This evidently occurs more frequently in those patients who suffer multiple trauma with or without CNS injury. Of the patients with only CNS injury it has been found that those with spinal cord trauma have higher gastrin levels than those with closed head injuries; concomitantly, decerebrate patients have higher gastrin levels than nondecerebrate patients.[4]

Proposed physiologic models for the production of ulcer include (1) parasympathetic-sympathetic mismatch (see section on "Innervation of the Bowel"), (2) disruption of the neuroendocrine axis with ACTH, corticosteroid, catecholamine release, and (3) paralytic vasodilatation resulting in hemorrhage and necrosis with consequent increased sensitivity to the actions of gastric acidity and enzyme production.

It is fair to say, however, that a definitive answer for the cause of gastroduodenal ulceration in quadriplegia has not yet been established.

Incidence of Ulcer

There is an impressive incidence of peptic ulceration in the immediate postinjury period. Figures such as 5% to 22% have been quoted.[6] In the chronic phase (beginning six months to one year after injury), there has been, at least in one study,[5] a higher incidence of erosion (11 out of 40) as compared to ulcer (two out of 40) as demonstrated by gastroscopy. Erosions are mainly gastric, and ulcers are mainly duodenal.

Perforation

As is the case in non–spinal-cord-injured patients, there is a higher incidence of perforation of duodenal as compared to gastric ulcers. As discussed previously, the symptoms of perforation fall into the "nonspecific" category, and include shoulder tip pain and the sensation of illness, nausea, and vomiting. Abdominal distention may be absent. There is increased abdominal wall spasticity and there are absent bowel sounds. Aside from the usual laboratory studies, abdominal x-rays are of the utmost importance. We have found there is a common tendency to do only supine films on quadriplegics in view of the difficulties encountered in sitting these patients up for any length of time, especially when they are ill. It is essential that an upright film after a few minutes of sitting be done in order to look for air under the diaphragm. If the patient cannot sit, a recumbent film with horizontal beam should be done, again after a few minutes of maintenance of the recumbent position. If these films are not done (and a diagnosis of perforation is not made) the patient may mistakenly be thought to have "gastroenteritis," fecal impaction, etc. Ongoing peritonitis (as will be discussed below) leads one further into the jungle of nonspecific GI tract symptoms in the quadriplegic. In one study, 10% of all acute mortalities was caused by gastrointestinal problems. Of these mortalities, the most common cause was perforation of a hollow viscus with peritonitis.

HEMORRHAGE

As is seen in other acute gastrointestinal entities in quadriplegia, GI tract hemorrhage can present in an occult way. The usual signs, such as postural hypotension or black stools, may be missing (the latter because of slower transit time), and tachycardia and hypotension may be misinterpreted because of the frequent incidence of these signs in other complications of quadriplegia. The presence of hematemesis is of course very helpful, but in hemorrhage from the duodenum or below this is much less common than in gastric or esophageal causes (erosive gastritis, gastric ulcer, esophageal erosion, and Mallory-Weiss syndrome).

In spinal cord injury, when associated with generalized trauma, especially penetrating or crush injury, there is an incidence of extraluminal, intra- or retroperitoneal hemorrhage, due to ruptured spleen, laceration of the kidney, or laceration of the liver. The diagnosis of these problems is even more difficult in the quadriplegic since the usual signs of hemorrhage are frequently absent.

There should be a high index of suspicion of occult intra-abdominal hemorrhage in the acutely injured spinal cord patient. As has been stated before,[6,7] gastroduodenal ulceration has a much higher incidence in the four to six weeks after injury than at any time later in the course of spinal cord injury. According to different studies,[6,8] the incidence of bleeding ulcer can range between 5% and 22% in the above time period. Duodenal ulcer has been described as more frequent than gastric ulcer in spinal cord injury patients.

In one study of 500 patients[6] it was found that the incidence of hemorrhage was equal in gastric and duodenal ulcer.

More common than ulcer is the occurrence of gastric erosions, which in one study[5] were five times more common than ulcer. The early symptoms associated with this entity are similar to those associated with ulcer, namely anorexia and nausea. It must be emphasized, however, that the diagnosis of gastric erosion is an endoscopic one, and therefore to all practical purposes the therapy of erosions and ulcer is identical.

In one study in symptomatic patients,[5] 19 of 40 patients had abnormal endoscopy findings. Of these, 11 patients had gastric erosions, six had hyperemic changes, and two had gastric ulcer. Of interest is the fact that in these patients there was no isolated duodenal involvement. In the patients who did have duodenal involvement duodenitis, duodenal erosions and ulcers were demonstrated in five patients.

PANCREATITIS

Pancreatitis has its highest incidence in the first month after trauma. The etiology of pancreatitis in quadriplegics without antecedent history of alcoholism or gall bladder disease is thought to be on the following bases: (1) spasm of the sphincter of Oddi, causing stasis of secretions[8]; (2) increased circulation of calcium (from immobility) causing direct activation of trypsinogen[9]; (3) the use of steroids causes increased viscosity of pancreatic secretions.

Pain is of course the hallmark of the presentation of pancreatitis in persons whose spinal cord is intact. The symptomatology of pancreatitis in spinal cord injury frequently includes fever and vomiting. Shoulder pain (so helpful in the diagnosis of perforated ulcer) is frequently absent, and the physical findings are limited to the absence or diminution of bowel sounds and of abdominal wall spasticity.

Increase of the serum urinary and peritoneal amylase level is present. As usual, amylase clearance is helpful even when the serum amylase value is normal but when the diagnosis is suspected. False elevation of the serum amylase level can be secondary to the use of codeine and morphine, which result in spasm of the sphincter of Oddi. In cases of multiple trauma, amylase elevation may be due to muscle trauma or to gut injury. Fractionation of the amylase will clarify this point and may show increase of other than alpha (pancreatic) amylase.

The treatment of pancreatitis in the spinal-cord-injured person is no different than in any other patient with this entity and need not be covered further here.

SUPERIOR MESENTERIC ARTERY (SMA) SYNDROME

The SMA syndrome is an entity in which the midtransverse duodenum is compressed by the superior mesenteric artery. Symptoms of duodenal obstruction such as postprandial vomiting of green material, distention, and abdominal discomfort are seen. Large amounts of bile-stained fluid are obtained on nasogastric intubation, and the abrupt cessation of the barium column in the third part of the duodenum is diagnostic when a GI series is performed.[10]

This syndrome has also been seen in patients placed in body casts, in those with severe weight loss, and in persons with spinal deformity.[10] In all these cases the angle between the aorta and the superior mesenteric artery becomes more acute either because of hyperlordosis or because of the supine position (particularly in the postprandial state). Loss of periduodenal areolar tissues secondary to severe weight loss has also been implicated in the etiology of this syndrome.[11]

In most cases the symptoms can be relieved by simple mechanical means. These include the use of (lumbosacral) corsets designed to relieve the hyperlordosis and to push the abdominal contents up. Upright position after meals and, in the long run, the regaining of lost weight are also helpful. In the unusual case, surgical measures such as duodenojejunostomy may have to be used if duodenal obstruction is not relieved by mechanical means.

APPENDICITIS

Acute appendicitis should be suspected as always in a differential diagnosis of symptoms related to the GI tract in spinal-cord-injured persons. Aside from the usual signs (such as abdominal distention) and symptoms (such as anorexia and nausea), the presence of fever and pain in the right iliac fossa and an increase in abdominal wall spasticity should alert the physician to the possibility of this diagnosis. The decision to explore the abdomen of a quadriplegic with the above constellation of symptoms and signs is not an easy one. Acute urinary tract infection, fecal impaction, and pelvic inflammatory disease in female patients all can mimic the already unclear picture of acute appendicitis in spinal-cord-injured patients. However, if the appropriate studies fail to reveal the existence of one of the above entities, then an exploratory laparotomy is indicated to forestall the septic complications of untreated acute appendicitis.

FECAL IMPACTION

It is the rare quadriplegic who does not at some time or another suffer from the sequelae of fecal impaction. Gore et al.[9] state that fecal impaction is the most common gastrointestinal complication of quadriplegia. Quadriplegics share with paraplegics the propensity to lower segment fecal impaction. However, an added problem for quadriplegics is fecal impaction as far up as the transverse colon. This added propensity is understandable in light of the previously discussed imbalance between sympathetic and parasympathetic stimuli in the quadriplegic, resulting in an ineffective peristaltic wave.

As is well known, fecal impaction frequently presents with diarrhea. The reason for this is that the fecal impaction acts as a partially obstructive mass resulting in oozing of liquid fecal material around the mass. Another presentation may be one in which gallbladder disease or ulcer may be mimicked in that the patient has had a vague upper abdominal discomfort. Autonomic hyperreflexia and fever, as well as anorexia and sense of fullness, may all be presenting clinical pictures of fecal impaction.

Physical examination is usually not very revealing. There may be some degree of abdominal distention. Bowel sounds may be diminished, normal, or increased. Rectal palpation of a large mass of hard stool, which is characteristic in fecal impaction in non–spinal-cord-injured persons as well as in paraplegics, may well not be present in quadriplegics with high impaction.

A bowel routine is initiated to ensure daily evacuation at a predictable time and to avoid soiling during active hours.

The patient takes stool softeners daily (e.g., Colace®). Natural fiber products such as senna can be added. At the time of desired evacuation a suppository (e.g., Therevac®) is used. Suppositories that may be irritating on a long-term basis (i.e., Dulcolax®) should be avoided on a daily schedule but may be used periodically.*

Evacuation is facilitated by using a bedside commode which

---

*Colace®, docusate sodium; Therevac®, disposable enema; Dulcolax®, bisacodyl.

adds the effect of gravity. A forceful Valsalva maneuver, which a quadriplegic patient cannot perform, is not necessary under these circumstances. Daily variations of the water and fiber intake can dramatically influence results. The patient's participation in a routine is important for it to be successful.

In summary, one should routinely suspect fecal impaction in quadriplegics who are not exposed to a daily bowel routine. The presence of the symptoms and signs enumerated above should alert the clinician to the presence of this frequent disorder.

REFERENCES

1. Tibbs P.A., Bivins B.A., Young A.B.: The problem of acute abdominal disease during spinal shock. *Am. Surg.* 6:366-368, 1979.
2. Tibbs P.A., Young A.B., Bivins B.A., et al.: Diagnosis of acute abdominal injuries in patients with spinal shock: Value of diagnostic peritoneal lavage. *J. Trauma,* 20:55-57, 1980.
3. Miller F., Fenzi T.C.: Prolonged ileus with acute spinal cord injury responding to metaclopramide. *Paraplegia* 19:43-45, 1981,
4. Bowen J.C., Flemming W.H., Thompsen J.C.: Increased gastrin release following penetrating central nervous system injury. *Surgery* 75:720-724, 1974.
5. Tanaka M., Uchiyama M., Kitano M.: Gastroduodenal disease in chronic spinal cord injuries. *Arch. Surg.* 114:185-187, 1979.
6. Kewalramani I.S.: Neurogenic gastroduodenal ulceration and bleeding associated with spinal cord injuries. *J. Trauma* 19:259-265, 1979.
7. Gore R.M., Mintzer R.A., Calenoff L.: Gastrointestinal complications of spinal cord injury. *Spine* 6:538-544, 1981.
8. Carey M.E., Nance F.C., Kirgis H.D., et al.: Pancreatitis following spinal cord injury. *J. Neurosurg.* 47:917-922, 1977.
9. Gore R.M., Mintzer R.A., Calenoff L.: Gastrointestinal complications of spinal cord injury. *Spine* 6:538-544, 1981.
10. Ramos M.: Recurrent superior mesenteric artery syndrome in a quadriplegic patient. *A.P.M.R.* 56:68-88, 1975.
11. Gore R.M., Mintzer R.A., Calenoff L.: Gastrointestinal complications of spinal cord injury. *Spine* 6:538-544, 1981.
12. Cannon R.A., Cox K.L.: Recurrent vomiting in a spastic quadriplegic. *Hosp. Pract.* March 1981, pp. 41-47.
13. Charney K.J., Juler G.L., Comarr A.E.: General surgery problems in patients with spinal cord injuries. *Arch. Surg.* 110:1083-1088, 1975.

14. Christy J.P.: Complications of combat casualties with combined injuries of bone and bowel: Personal experience with nineteen patients. *Surgery* 72:270–274, 1972.
15. Claus-Walker J., Halstead L.S.: Autonomic drugs in spinal cord injury: Temporal prescription profile. *A.P.M.R.* 59:363-367, 1978.
16. Connell A.M., Paeslack V., Frankel H.L.: The physiology and pathophysiology of constipation. Papers read at the 1966 Scientific Meeting. *Paraplegia,* pp. 244-458.
17. Devroede G., Arban P., Gugvay C., et al.: Traumatic constipation. *Gastroenterology* 77:1258-1266, 1979.
18. Djergaian R.S., Staas W.E.: Upper gastrointestinal bleeding in a quadriplegic patient. *A.P.M.R.* 62:345-346, 1981.
19. Dollfus P., Holdenbach G.L., Husser J.M., et al.: Must appendicitis be still considered as a rare complication in quadriplegia? *Paraplegia* 11:306-309, 1973.
20. Epstein N., Hood D.C., Ransohoff J.: Gastrointestinal bleeding in patients with spinal cord trauma. *J. Neurosurg.* 54:16-20, 1981.
21. Green B.A., Green K.L., Klose K.J.: Kinetic nursing for acute spinal cord injury patients. *Paraplegia* 18:181-186, 1980.
22. Hackler R.H.: A 25-year prospective mortality study in the spinal cord injured patient: Comparison with the long-term living paraplegic. *J. Urol.* 117:486-488, 1977.
23. Larkin J., Moylan J.: Priorities in management of trauma victims. *Crit. Care Med.* 3:192-195, 1975.
24. McSweeney T.: The early management of associated injuries in the presence of co-incident damage to the spinal cord. Papers read at the 1967 Scientific Meeting at Stoke Mandeville Hospital, Aylesbury, July 27–29, 1967. *Paraplegia* pp. 189-209.
25. Meshkinpour H., Nouroozi F., Glick M.E.: Colonic compliance in patients with spinal cord injury. *A.P.M.R.* 64:111-112, 1983.
26. Lipschitz R.: Associated injuries and complications of stab wounds of the spinal cord. *Paraplegia* pp. 75-82.
27. Miller L.S., Staas W.E., Herbison G.J.: Abdominal problems in patients with spinal cord lesions. *A.P.M.R.* 56:405-408, 1975.
28. Nelson R.P., Brugh R.: Bilateral ureteral obstruction secondary to massive fecal impaction. *Neurology* 16:403-406, 1980.
29. Osteen P.T., Ravsamian E.M.: Delayed gastric emptying after vagotomy and drainage in the spinal cord injury patient. *Paraplegia* 19:46-49, 1981.
30. O'Connor J.R.: Traumatic quadriplegia—a comprehensive review. *J. Rehabil.* May-June 1971, pp. 14-20.
31. Stanley W.G.: Follow-up care of the spinal cord injury patient. *A.F.P.* 24:105-107, 1981.

32. Steicher F.M.: The emergency management of the severely injured. *J. Trauma* 12:786-790, 1972.
33. Sutton R.A., MacPhail F., Bentley R., et al.: Acute gastric dilatation as a relatively late complication of tetraplegia due to very high cervical cord injury. *Paraplegia* 19:17-19, 1981.
34. Taylor R.G.: Spinal cord injury: Its many complications. *A.F.P.* 8:138-146, 1973.
35. Tudor L.L.: Bladder and bowel retraining. *Am. J. Nurs.* 70:2391-2393, 1970.
36. Walsh J.J., Nuseibch I., El-Masri W.: Perforated peptic ulcer in paraplegia. *Paraplegia* 11:310-313, 1974.
37. Watson N.: Late ileus in paraplegia. *Paraplegia* 19:13-16, 1981.
38. Wilson T.H.: Penetrating trauma of colon, cava, and cord. *J. Trauma* 16:411-413, 1976.

9

Musculoskeletal Complications

HETEROTOPIC OSSIFICATION and spasticity and, ultimately, muscle contractures are the main complications of quadriplegia as regards the musculoskeletal system.

Although not life threatening, the limitation of range of motion of the extremities can lead to severe functional impairment that inhibits the usual rehabilitation process. The medical aspects of these complications have increased in importance in recent years with advancing knowledge of both pathophysiology and therapy.

HETEROTOPIC OSSIFICATION

Heterotopic ossification is an entity of unknown etiology that involves the soft tissues below the level of the neurologic lesion. It can occur as soon as 19 days after injury and as late as several years after injury. This has sometimes also been referred to as *myositis ossificans*, but this is not actually correct. Myositis ossificans is an entity that is either congenital or posttraumatic in origin. The latter involves ossification usually in muscles at sites of displaced periostum with (usually) hematoma formation. The congenital variety does not involve trauma and is not associated with hematoma.

Heterotopic ossification is secondary to an unknown stimulus in which there is an inflammation of extra-articular soft tissue with subsequent deposition of cancellous bone. The usual presentation is that of fever, local warmth, and swelling with subsequent limited range of motion and, ultimately, with ankylosis. The incidence of this condition does not depend on the presence or absence of spasticity. The most common sites of occurrence of heterotopic ossification are the hips, knees, elbows, and shoulders, and occasionally there is involvement of the spine and hands.

It is obvious that the appearance of unusual warmth, swelling, and tenderness in any extremity in the immobilized patient should make the clinician suspicious of deep venous thrombosis. A negative Doppler study finding in this situation should suggest the very real possibility of the heterotopic ossification.

Within the first ten days of the formation of heterotopic ossification, the plain x-ray films of the affected area are usually negative. At this stage, however, the bone scan is usually already positive, showing evidence of bone formation in the affected soft tissues. In the early stages, the bone alkaline phosphatase level and erythrocyte sedimentation rate (ESR) usually is elevated and remains elevated as the condition matures. As time goes on and evidence of local inflammation subsides, the alkaline phosphatase concentration begins to diminish and the bone scan activity begins to approach normal. Thus, a stable area of ossification is left in the affected soft tissues.

The management of heterotopic ossification is oriented to multiple factors: (1) alleviation of diminished range of motion, and (2) control of decubiti arising from the pressure of soft tissue superimposed on a bony prominence (the area of heterotopic ossification). Heterotopic ossification is a significant complication of spinal cord injury. Twenty percent of all spinal cord injury patients can incur this complication,[1] and 3% of all spinal cord injury patients ultimately have ankylosis secondary to this condition.

The most common complication of heterotopic ossification is diminished range of motion. There is a 3% incidence of bony ankylosis in the patients with diminished range of motion.[1] The maintenance of adequate range of motion is therefore of paramount importance. Active and passive range of motion exercise may be continued after the diagnosis of heterotopic ossification has been made. There is no evidence to suggest that range of motion exercise in any way accelerates the process. In fact, much of the literature implies that interruption of motion may facilitate the progression from diminished range of motion to ankylosis.

As is the case in pressure of soft tissue on bony prominences with ultimate development of decubiti, areas of heterotopic ossification can act in the same way. Therefore, persistent pressure sores resistant to usual forms of therapy occurring especially in the areas of high risk for heterotopic ossification (hips, knees, etc.) should alert the physician to the possibility of underlying heterotopic ossification. The presence of a unilateral decubitus at the ischium should alert the clinician to the possible presence of heterotopic ossification. By limiting the range of motion at the hip, the arc of the sitting position is changed; there is consequently increased pressure on one ischium with resultant breakdown.

THERAPY

The maintenance of adequate range of motion is usually sufficient as palliation for this condition. There are two main indications for surgical excision of these bony lesions: (1) the persistence of decubitus ulcer, and (2) nonreversible and progressive limitation of range of motion with consequent functional impairment. The procedure involves excision of the areas of new bone formation. Rotation of a flap depends on the area involved and the condition of the overlying skin.

Disodium editronate diphosphonate is a pyrophosphate-like drug used to prevent mineralization by blocking tranformation or amorphous calcium phosphate into crystalline hydroxy apatite. Its great advantage is that it accumulates only in bone and that it is not metabolized and is excreted unchanged in the urine. As far as its use in heterotopic ossification is concerned, there are two principal modes of therapy. One has been an attempt to prevent new bone formation after areas of heterotopic ossification have been removed surgically; the other involves prophylactic treatment of spinal cord injury patients with this drug. In both forms of therapy encouraging results have been encountered.

OSTEOPOROSIS

Diffuse osteoporosis usually begins to occur radiologically in spinal cord injury patients after approximately six months. In light of current knowledge, it is evident that osteoporosis can be detected earlier by means of computed tomography (CT).[3] CT density measurements can pick up 2% to 3% bone loss and can specifically detect trabecular bone loss. This is important because current studies involving osteoporosis patients and spinal-cord-injured patients show that trabecular bone is more involved than cortical bone.

The clinical reports of osteoporosis in quadriplegia are open to question. Its incidence is probably under-reported if it is based on clinical observation. Since pain is not perceived and spontaneous motion is very limited, the only significant clinical events that occur in this condition are kyphosis secondary to anterior wedge fractures and other fractures resulting from accidental falls. Occasionally extremity fractures occur, chiefly as a result of transfer activities. In the patient with neurologically incomplete lesions, conservative management consisting of splinting with intermittent ranging is usually more than adequate therapy. As further research is done more clinical applications may become clear.

OSTEOMYELITIS

This is usually seen in the quadriplegic secondary either to an infection at the site of the original trauma or as a result of extension of the decubitus ulcer to bone with soft-tissue abscess formation. In these settings, the diagnosis of osteomyelitis is based on the usual criteria. In a setting of either recent trauma or known decubiti, the presence of fever, elevated sedimentation rate, nonhealing decubiti, as well as suggestive x-ray and/or CT scan changes, a diagnosis of osteomyelitis should be considered.

SPINAL DEFORMITY

In preadolescent quadriplegics who have had spinal cord injury before full skeletal maturation has been achieved, there is the risk of spinal deformity later in the course. The reason for this is because of the muscle imbalance that can continue to be a deforming force even after skeletal maturity has occurred.

In general, in all quadriplegics, excessive lordosis, kyphosis, and scoliosis are commonly seen. The change in the curve of the spine and any associated thoracic rotation can lead to a change in sitting balance. This in turn redistributes pressure in the sitting position and can lead to ischial, thoracic, or midline decubitus ulcers, depending on the forces present.

As in other forms of spinal deformity with a neuromuscular component, the deforming force goes on beyond full skeletal maturity. With progression of the spinal curvature, progressive changes in pulmonary function occur. The pattern of respiratory disturbance in these patients is of the restrictive variety. Forced expiratory flow volume loops are extremely helpful in the diagnosis of this disturbance and should be included in pulmonary function testing if this entity is suspected.

MUSCLE

Spasticity is defined as involuntary muscle activity resulting from an interruption of the inhibiting pathways of the spinal reflex arc. It is a major clinical problem in spinal cord injury patients. If it is not suppressed it encourages development of contractures because of difficulty in the performance of ranging exercises. Often the physician will observe flinging motions of the arms or legs, which may appear voluntary. These are in fact involuntary movements caused by muscle contraction, and the patient is unable to control them. On clinical examination, increased muscle tone giving way to resistance, and clonus are indications of spasticity. During the period of spinal shock, patients are flaccid. Spasticity usually begins to appear about six weeks after injury and can be treated with oral medications. Drugs commonly used are diazepam, baclofen, and dantrolene sodium.

Dantrolene sodium once enjoyed a vogue in the therapy of spasticity. It acts by direct effect on the contractile mechanism of skeletal muscle without interfering with cardiac muscle, smooth muscle, neural pathways, or the neuromuscular junction. The current hypothesis is that it inhibits the release of calcium from the sarcoplasmic reticulum. This type of drug would seem to be ideal for the treatment of spasticity and indeed has been used with good effect. However, there have been reports of deaths due to hepatotoxicity in patients taking the drug for more than 60 days. The early sign of toxicity is elevation of the SGOT, with ultimate development of jaundice. The safeguards used in this setting are performance of weekly liver function studies and the avoidance of usage of the drug for more than 60 days, since the effect of long-term therapy has not been established in humans. In animal studies, cardiac and smooth muscle are unaffected by the drug, but it has been recommended that it not be used in the presence of cardiac disease and chronic obstructive pulmonary disease. Obviously, the drug should not be used in the presence of preexisting hepatic disease.

Another drug used for the suppression of muscle spasticity is diazepam (Valium®), whose actions comprise effects on the limbic system, thalamus, and hypothalamus (in animal studies). Although it is usually used for its calmative effects, it can be used for the relief of spasticity. In many centers it is the first-line drug used for spasticity. The dosage used is highly variable, but it is our practice to start patients on approximately 10 mg/day and to raise the dosage to as high as 40 mg/day. Although spasticity frequently diminishes during treatment with this drug, the side effects make continuation of therapy with the drug difficult. Sedation and ultimate depression are limiting factors that may be so disabling that the drug has to be discontinued.

The medication frequently used as a replacement for diazepam is baclofen. Its definitive mode of action is unknown, but it is thought to inhibit postsynaptic reflexes at the spinal level. The current concept is that this is accomplished by increased polarization of the afferent terminals. The advantage of this drug is that it causes less drowsiness than diazepam and therefore is less likely to be abused. Also, in contrast to diazepam, it does not cause psychic or physical dependence per se. However, hallucinations and seizures have been described with sudden withdrawal from high dosage. Occasionally, confusion, headaches, and GI tract upset have been described with the use of this drug.

All in all, the lack of consistent efficacy of the oral drugs coupled with multiplicity of side effects speak to the fact that a definitive drug for treatment of spasticity has not yet been found. For any other modalities used, however, an adequate trial of oral medication with appropriate time given to equilibrate on a given dose should be given.

If drug therapy has not been found to be beneficial, it is our custom to resort to the use of selective nerve blocks. These are of two types: short-acting, and so-called permanent block. The short-acting nerve block is utilized mainly for diagnostic reasons. Lidocaine, which has an evanescent effect (one to two hours), is injected. During this period the efficacy on spasticity is evaluated. These one to two hours will be utilized for aggressive manipulation which differentiates between spasticity (area in question can be moved during the block) and fixation of bone or soft tissue (area cannot be moved during the block). It is also possible to gauge the amount of deformity present that may be either on the basis of bone ankylosis or soft-tissue sclerosis. A temporary block is therefore of use in the evaluation of patients for surgical procedures such as tendon release, tendon transfer, or excision of heterotopic ossification.

Permanent block is effective for six months or longer. Phenol is the agent of choice. Blocks may be done by direct injection of the nerve or motor point. These blocks must be performed under carefully controlled circumstances because accidental IV injection of phenol can lead to massive coagulopathy. Electrodiagnostic monitoring should be used, so that the injection can be performed at exactly the desired site. It may be necessary to repeat the block at any time from six months to years after the initial procedure. A properly performed block should not result in motor weakness. It should be remembered that those patients who depend on spasticity for ambulation may lose some functional ground. This should not be construed as a complication of the nerve block.

Repeated intramuscular or IV injections should be avoided in patients with paralyzed musculature. The venous drainage in these muscles is poor and any extravasation is poorly cleared. In the same context, any intramuscular material will be poorly absorbed, thus increasing the likelihood of loculation of fluid and subsequent abscess formation.

REFERENCES

1. Hernandez A.M., Fjorner J.V., De la Fuente T., et al.: The para-articular ossifications in our paraplegics and tetraplegics: A survey of 704 patients. *Paraplegia* 16:272-275, 1978.
2. Stover S., Niemann K.M.W., Miller J.M.: Disodium etidronate in the prevention of postoperative recurrence of heterotopic ossification in spinal cord injury patients. *J. Bone Joint Surg.* 58-A:683–688, 1976.
3. Bedbrook G.M., Edibam R.C.: The study of spinal deformity in traumatic spinal paralysis. *Paraplegia* 10:321-225, 1978.
4. Griffiths H.J., Bushueff B., Zimmerman R.E.: Investigation of the loss of bone mineral in patients with spinal cord injury. *Paraplegia* 14:207-212, 1976.
5. Malik G.M., Sapico F.L., Montgomerie J.Z.: Severe vertebral osteomyelitis in patients with spinal cord injury. *Ann. Intern. Med.* 142:807-808, 1982.
6. Hassard G.H.: Heterotopic bone formation about the hip and unilateral decubitus ulcers in spinal cord injury. *A.P.M.R.* 56:355-358, 1975.
7. Lancourt J.E., Dickson J.H., Carter R.E.: Paralytic spinal deformity following traumatic spinal cord injury in children and adolescents. *J. Bone Joint Surg.* 63-A:47-53, 1981.
8. Mayfield J.K., Erkkila J.C., Winter R.B.: Spine deformity subsequent to acquired childhood spinal cord injury. *J. Bone Joint Surg.* 63-A:1401-1411, 1981.
9. Ohry A., Shemesh Y., Zak R., et al.: Zinc and osteoporosis in patients with spinal cord injury. *Paraplegia* 18:174-180, 1980.
10. Wharton G.W., Morgan T.H.: Ankylosis in the paralyzed patient. *J. Bone Joint Surg.* 52-A:105-112, 1970.

10

Deep Venous Thrombosis and Thromboembolism

DEEP VENOUS THROMBOSIS is a relatively frequent phenomenon in quadriplegics, with a 12% to 20% incidence reported in some studies.[1] Most of the cases occur in the first two to three weeks after injury. Pulmonary embolism occurs in approximately 5% of quadriplegics, again usually within the first two to three weeks after injury. Deep venous thrombosis is more common in quadriplegics than in paraplegics, and is more common in patients with cervical lesions of the cord. It is certainly more common in the patient with a neurologically complete motorsensory involvement.

Through I121-labeled fibrinogen studies it has been found that organized thrombosis of calf veins appears as early as 36 hours after injury. Trauma itself is of course a major stimulus to the activation of the clotting system.[2,3]

Either at the time of injury or during spinal operations subsequent to the injury, tissue thromboplastin is released, causing activation of the extrinsic pathway via factor VII. In addition, levels of factor VIII, which is produced by endothelial cells, have been found to rise dramatically after spinal cord injury. Persistently high levels of factor VIII have been correlated with the development of deep venous thrombosis. Since this factor is involved in platelet adhesiveness, it may be responsible for some of the increased incidence of thrombosis in these patients by causing recruitment of greater numbers of platelets to the site of the vascular injury or to the propagating clot.

CLINICAL PICTURE OF DEEP VENOUS THROMBOSIS

In the non-neurologically impaired individual, deep venous thrombosis and pulmonary embolism frequently present in an occult way. In recent years, the diagnosis of pulmonary embolism has been made on the basis of more and more occult clinical presentations in the setting of technologically more sophisticated laboratory substantiation. Unexplained fever or cough, breathlessness at rest and/or exercise, unexplained electrocardiographic (ECG) changes all have been seen more and more as the only presenting factors in pulmonary embolism.

The "classic" presentation of hemoptysis and pleuritic chest pain appears to be much less frequent than the more "occult" signs enumerated above. In the quadriplegic, in whom other serious intercurrent problems present in an unusual way, pulmonary embolus and deep venous thrombosis are no exception. Whereas in the non spinal cord injured individual, pain is the presenting complaint in deep venous thrombosis, painless leg swelling is the rule in the deep venous thrombosis of quadriplegics. Leg edema in quadriplegics may also be due to subcutaneous abscess due to pressure sores or hematoma secondary to previous trauma. These conditions may be readily diagnosed by the clinical examination and by computerized scanning and/or ultrasound. In the absence of evidence for the above conditions, deep venous thrombosis, which is probably the most common cause of leg edema in quadriplegics, must be considered to be the cause until proven otherwise.

Cachexia and muscle atrophy in the lower extremities distort the "normal" appearance of the calf and thigh. By visual inspection alone, therefore, edema cannot be diagnosed reliably in all cases. Obvious unilateral enlargement of an extremity is of course a reliable sign, but the earlier manifestations of deep venous thrombosis (which is most usually unilateral) may be missed by the usual brief clinical inspection.

We therefore recommend daily routine measurement of thighs and calves for the three weeks postinjury. Measurements should of course be carried out at any other time in case deep venous thrombosis is suspected for any other reason.

In the patient with spinal cord injury the measurement of objective signs of deep venous thrombosis is essential since pain is not experienced, edema may be occult, and Homans' sign is usually not elicitable. The Doppler ultrasound flow detector maneuver has proven to be very helpful in the diagnosis of deep venous thrombosis. However, the Doppler study is only positive if at least 50% of the affected vessel has been occluded.[4] Its advantage is the possibility of performing the test as an emergency procedure (even at the bedside) and the ease and rapidity with which it can be performed.

Impedance plethysmography is another noninvasive procedure for the detection of lower extremity deep venous thrombosis. It is technically more difficult than the Doppler. Its use is mainly in the detection of large clots; therefore calf venous obstruction is not accurately diagnosed by this method.

I 121 scanning has been found to have as high as 100% accuracy in one study.[5] However, it does not lend itself to emergency situations because of the intrinsically complicated nature of the procedure. This is used primarily as a research tool and is of very little use in acute clinical conditions.[4] However, there is definitely a place for scanning in the diagnosis of chronic venous disease, a situation in which the use of impedance plethysmography and Doppler testing are of lesser use.

I 121 injection into the foot is helpful in delineating the venous circulation in patients with chronic venous disease and suspected recurrence of deep venous thrombosis. Technetium, or Tc-labeled human albumin has also been used in outlining the venous system. An added advantage in using this material is the potential for simultaneous lung scanning, so that both deep venous thrombosis and pulmonary embolism can be searched for with one injection.

Since the advent of noninvasive procedures, the use of venography in diagnosis of deep venous thrombosis has declined. The disadvantages of this procedure are the use of dye (with potential for allergic reaction, or nephrotoxicity) and the incidence of infiltration of the material. Occasionally, however, it is of use if noninvasive tests are equivocal and if there is a very real potential danger to empirical anticoagulation. In view of the generally low incidence of diagnosis of deep venous thrombosis by clinical means alone, it has been suggested that a routine Doppler test be performed in patients who are at risk for this complication of trauma and/or severe illness.[4] We can thus extrapolate to spinal-cord-injured patients the suggestion that routine Doppler testing of the lower extremities be done on a weekly basis for the first month after injury. This is especially important since, as stated above, 80% of all deep venous thrombosis and pulmonary embolism occur during this time.

As has been suggested, the diagnosis of pulmonary embolism is frequently based on the proper appreciation by the clinician of disparate signs and symptoms. This is especially true in the quadriplegic. Transient episodes of shortness of breath, feelings of chest compression, unexplained fever and/or tachycardia, and cough (either nonproductive or productive of mucoid and/or sanguinous material) are all clues to the existence of pulmonary embolism. Deep venous thrombosis may be apparent clinically but may only be diagnosable by the means enumerated above. In some instances, whatever the procedures utilized, thromboembolism may not be detectable. Certainly in a bedridden inactive population, any clinical sign out of the ordinary, especially if it relates to the chest, should make the clinician suspicious of the existence of a pulmonary embolus. As far as substantiation of the diagnosis is concerned, the lung scan has had a significant degree of accuracy. The addition in recent years of the ventilation scan in addition to the perfusion scan has increased the accuracy of this procedure even further.

Infiltrates on chest x-ray, evidence of new right axis deviation or right bundle branch block on ECG, and new elevation of the lactic dehydrogenase (LDH) level all are secondary criteria in this diagnosis and should not be relied on unduly. Arterial oxygen desaturation goes along with pulmonary embolism but does not offer definitive diagnostic implications.

Pulmonary angiography is, again, used sparingly. It is occasionally complicated by sudden death, dye reactions, and requires extensive setup procedures. However, in patients who are at very real risk for complications of anticoagulation (active peptic ulcer, current bleeding from another site, etc.) angiography can be very helpful in the definitive diagnosis of pulmonary artery obstruction.

THERAPY OF THROMBOEMBOLISM

THE THERAPY OF DEEP VEIN THROMBOSIS

In a high-risk population in which there is no spontaneous leg movement and in which there is prolonged bedrest as well, it is essential to prevent deep vein thrombosis of the lower extremities before a possibly catastrophic episode of pulmonary embolism can develop. It has been shown[6] that prompt initiation of small-dose heparin therapy (mini-heparin) as soon as possible after injury has been related to decreased incidence of pulmonary embolism. These small amounts of heparin are not sufficient for true anticoagulation, and normal partial thromboplastin times are maintained throughout. The effect of the mini-heparin therapy is felt to be on the basis of inhibition of activation of factor X with consequent slowing down of the coagulation cascade.

Although good results have been obtained with full anticoagulation with oral anticoagulants,[7] the current usual practice, especially in the United States, is to administer low-dose heparin, usually 5,000 units subcutaneously every 12 hours. Several schedules have been described: (1) subcutaneous heparin started right after injury and continued for three months; (2) subcutaneous heparin started after injury, but in obese patients or patients with previous deep vein thrombosis, heparin is continued for six months; (3) heparin therapy is started after injury but discontinued as soon as the patient is started in the wheelchair. In several studies dealing with small numbers of patients, the incidence of deep vein thrombosis in patients treated with mini-heparin[8] or mini-heparin for the first month and coumadin for the next two months was significantly reduced.

Aspirin is sometimes used along with mini-heparin for its inhibitory effect on platelet aggregation. However, its effect in prevention of thrombosis in a low-pressure immobilized limb has not been clarified.

Our practice is to use mini-heparin for at least three months after injury. Range of motion therapy and anti-embolism stockings should also be used in an attempt to prevent venous thrombosis.

If deep venous thrombosis supervenes, full-scale anticoagulation with heparin with an initial loading dose with subsequent administration of a continuous drip and monitored by partial thromboplastin times should be undertaken.

In the quadriplegic, several cautions must be observed: Warm soaks to the affected leg should not be used. Since this is in any case not therapeutic but just pain relieving, it is better to dispense with it in an individual who has no pain perception; patients may inadvertently be burned, and the risk of this is not outweighed by the therapeutic potential of soaks. Range of motion exercises are contraindicated for at least the first 72 hours after the diagnosis of deep vein thrombosis is made. In addition, excessive manipulation of the extremity should be avoided since it may cause dislodgement of the thrombus and thus cause embolization.

The duration of full-scale heparinization is variable. It is our practice to administer heparin for at least ten days. Around the seventh day of heparinization, coumadin administration is begun. A therapeutic level of prothrombin time should then be present around the tenth day of heparin therapy. Heparin should not be discontinued, however, until the prothrombin time is therapeutic, which is 1½ to two times control. The length of therapy with coumadin is variable; there is no hard and fast rule. We usually keep patients with first episodes of deep vein thrombosis anticoagulated for three months. Recurrence of deep venous thrombosis and evidence of chronic deep vein stasis are considerations for more prolonged and, in some cases, even permanent anticoagulation.

Many drugs interact with oral anticoagulants. Care should be taken to consider interaction with drugs that the patient is already taking when treatment with anticoagulants is begun. Table 10–1 demonstrates some of the most important drug interactions.[10]

Anticoagulant-induced bleeding may present in a nonapparent manner in all individuals. Retroperitoneal hematoma, bleeding into a large soft tissue space such as the thigh, in short any hemorrhage into a nonluminal space may present with hypotension, tachycardia, and anemia. Gastrointestinal tract hemorrhage may of course be more apparent, but in its early stages, as discussed in the chapter on gastrointestinal complications, it may be much more occult in the quadriplegic.

Occult bleeding must always be considered in the differential diagnosis of unexplained changes in the blood pressure and heart rate, even before there are changes in blood count. In a quadriplegic receiving anticoagulants this must be considered even more strongly. We suggest that the patient receiving oral anticoagulants have daily testing of prothrombin times, hematocrit readings every other day, and tests of stool for blood and urine for blood several times a week. Bleeding, al-

TABLE 10–1.–Drug Interference With Oral Anticoagulants*

DRUG	MECHANISM OF INTERFERENCE	RESULTS
Phenobarbital	Increased microsomal enzyme	Inhibition
Chloral hydrate	activity in the liver	
Meprobamate	Increased metabolic	
Glutethimide (Doriden®)	degradation of AC	
Haloperidol (Haldol®)		
Phenyramidol (Analexin®)	Inhibited metabolic degradation	Potentiation
Phenylbutazone (Butazolidin®)	Prevention of protein-binding	Potentiation
Oxyphenbutazone (Tandearil®)	peak levels of AC increased	
Diphenylhydantoin (Dilantin®)		
Salicylates (Aspirin®)		
Tetracyclines	Inhibited bacterial synthesis of	Potentiation
Neomycin	vitamin K	
Sulfisoxazole		
Clofibrate (Atromid®)	Unknown	Potentiation

*From Hachen H.J.: *Paraplegia* 12:176-187, 1974. Reprinted with permission.

though much more likely in a patient with a prothrombin time outside the therapeutic range, may be seen with a therapeutic prothrombin time as well. One should not be led away from a diagnosis of anticoagulant-induced bleeding by the level of the prothrombin time or the absence of evidence of luminal bleeding.

TREATMENT OF PULMONARY EMBOLUS

There has been a substantial decrease in the incidence of pulmonary embolization in quadriplegics treated with mini-heparin.[8] However, therapy with mini-heparin is not universal, and there is a well-known incidence of pulmonary embolus despite prophylactic heparin therapy. In addition, the incidence of embolization from deep venous thrombosis of the thigh is significantly higher than that with thrombosis confined to the infrapopliteal area. Therefore, the patient with proximal venous thrombosis must be watched even more closely for signs of pulmonary embolus.

Pulmonary embolus may of course be seen in the setting of obvious deep vein thrombosis. However, pulmonary embolus is frequently seen without overt existing or antecedent deep vein thrombosis. In some cases the diagnosis of deep vein thrombosis is made retrospectively, at the time of diagnosis of the pulmonary embolus. When pulmonary embolus is diagnosed, the patient immediately undergoes therapeutic (that is, full-scale) anticoagulation with heparin. As in the treatment of deep vein thrombosis, the initial loading dose is followed by continuous infusion under monitoring of the partial thromboplastin time (PTT). After ten days, and with coumadin therapy having been started several days before, heparin treatment is discontinued if there is a therapeutic level of prothrombin time. Again, the length of the administration of coumadin is variable. In many centers, the period of three to six months is usual.

Recent literature[9] has suggested that the efficacy of low-dose coumadin administration with prothrombin times only several seconds off control is the same as that with prothrombin times

1½ to two times off control. Thus it may be possible to keep patients on long-term anticoagulation therapy with prothrombin time determinations every one to two weeks and with the concomitantly decreased incidence of untoward bleeding.

Any patient taking anticoagulants should have stool and urine studies for blood and hematocrit readings twice weekly. After a predictable level of prothrombin time is obtained with a certain dose of coumadin, prothrombin time determinations may be obtained as infrequently as every one or two weeks. The same precautions described previously as far as development of interactions with coumadin are concerned should again be considered.

Despite full-scale, meticulous anticoagulation, some patients will have recurrence of pulmonary embolization. This group includes patients who are older, obese, and with associated illnesses such as cancer, or patients with a history of chronic venous disease with propagation of clot into the vena cava. These individuals will require mechanical interruption of the vena cava by umbrella placement, which can currently be done percutaneously, thus sparing an already ill patient an abdominal operation.

REFERENCES

1. Brach B.B.: Venous thrombosis in acute spinal cord paralysis. *J. Trauma* 17:289-292, 1977.
2. Silver J.R.: The prophylactic use of anticoagulant therapy in the prevention of pulmonary emboli in one hundred consecutive spinal injury patients. *Paraplegia* 12:188-196, 1974.
3. Raphael, Bruce, personal communication.
4. Barnes R.W.: Current status of noninvasive tests in the diagnosis of venous disease. *Surg. Clin. North Am.* 62:489-500, 1982.
5. Todd J.W.: Deep venous thrombosis in acute spinal cord injury: A comparison of ^{125}I fibrinogen leg scanning, impedance plethysmography and venography. *Paraplegia* 14:50-57, 1976.
6. Watson N.: Anti-coagulant therapy in the prevention of venous thrombosis and pulmonary embolism in the spinal cord injury. *Paraplegia* 16:265-269, 1978.
7. El Masri W.S., Silver J.R.: Prophylactic anticoagulant therapy in patients with spinal cord injury. *Paraplegia* 19:334-342, 1981.
8. Casas E.R., Sanchez M.P., Arias C.R., et al.: Prophylaxis of venous

thrombosis and pulmonary embolism in patients with acute traumatic spinal cord lesions. *Paraplegia* 15:209-214, 1977.

9. Hull R., Hirsh J., Jay R., et al.: Different intensities of oral anticoagulant therapy in the treatment of proximal-vein thrombosis. *N. Engl. J. Med.* 307:1676, 1982.

10. Hachen H.J.: Anticoagulant therapy in patients with spinal cord injury. *Paraplegia* 12:176-187, 1974.

11. Casas E.R., Sanchez M.P., Arias C.R., et al.: Prophylaxis of venous thrombosis and pulmonary embolism in patients with acute traumatic spinal cord lesions. *Paraplegia* 14:178-183, 1976.

12. Dollfus P. et al.: The value of the thromboelastogram as means of monitoring the sub-cutaneous preventive action of calcium heparinate. *Paraplegia* 18:157-166, 1980.

13. Frisbie J.H., Sasahara A.A.: Low-dose heparin prophylaxis for deep venous thrombosis in acute spinal cord injury patients: A controlled study. *Paraplegia* 19:343-346, 1981.

14. Naso F.: Pulmonary embolism in acute spinal cord injury. *A.P.M.R.* 55:257-278, 1974.

15. Perkash A., et al.: Experience with the management of thromboembolism in patients with spinal cord injury: I. Incidence, diagnosis and role of some risk factors. *Paraplegia* 16:322-331, 1978.

16. Perkash A.: Experience with the management of deep vein thrombosis in patients with spinal cord injury. *Paraplegia* 18:2-14, 1980.

17. Silver J.R.: Prophylactic anticoagulant therapy against pulmonary emboli in acute paraplegia. *Br. Med. J.* 2:338-340, 1970.

18. Van Hove E.: Prevention of thrombophlebitis in spinal injury patients. *Paraplegia* 16:332-335, 1978.

19. Watson N.: Venous thrombosis and pulmonary embolism in spinal cord injury. *Paraplegia* 5:113-121, 1967.

11

Decubitus Ulcers and Other Skin Problems

DECUBITUS ULCER FORMATION is one of the persistent problems in the care of quadriplegics. In one study[1] it has been estimated that up to 60% of patients with cervical cord injury can develop pressure sores during the acute post-traumatic period. The incidence is higher in quadriplegia than in paraplegia, and in complete lesions more than in incomplete lesions. Decubiti are more likely to be multiple than single. Occasionally, because of the circumstances of the injury or the method of transportation, decubiti are already present when the patient comes to medical attention.

Superficially, the decubitus ulcer problem may appear both minor and surgical in nature. However, anyone with experience in the care of spinal cord injury patients knows that even the most harmless-appearing pressure sore can have multiple debilitating complications, which can even terminate in the death of the patient.

Although surgery certainly has its place in the treatment of pressure sores, the major mode of therapy is really medical. Prevention and diagnosis of decubital tracking, therapy of secondary sepsis, and evaluation of remote complications (amyloidosis, osteomyelitis, etc.) all fall within the realm of the internist.

At this point it may well be worthwhile to briefly discuss the pathophysiology of pressure-related necrosis. Although it has been thought for many years that pressure sores begin as a skin abrasion, in recent times it has been shown that the ischemic process is primary and begins in the subcutaneous layers. Subcutaneous fat, although very compressible, has low tensile strength. It is very susceptible to vascular compromise. Shear stresses set up a mechanical force that allows angulation of the cutaneous vessels to occur, leading to ischemia. Any pressure over 30 mm Hg will allow this to occur. Sitting results in a pressure of more than 300 mm Hg, and even the most sophisticated relief cushions can only decrease the pressure by 100 to 200 mm Hg.

The other factor to be considered is of course the length of time that the pressure is exerted.[2] Hyperemia can start within 30 to 60 minutes, ischemia after two to six hours, and necrosis in over six hours of continuous pressure. Pressure sores are usually seen over bony prominences. Soft tissue overlying the bone is thus compressed between external pressure and the unyielding bone, thus compressing vascular supply. The most common bony prominences involved in pressure sores are, in descending order of frequency, (1) sacrum, (2) ischial areas, (3) trochanteric areas, (4) heels, (5) interspinous recesses, and (6) scalp (in patients with halo traction).

As stated previously, hyperemia is the first stage of pressure-related vascular change. This is reversible with the relief of pressure. If pressure is not released, the next stage is ischemia. Subcutaneous fat is most vulnerable to ischemic changes. Deep fascia is relatively resistant to vascular compromise and is more fixed than the subcutaneous layer; therefore, mechanical stress can lead to separation of the two layers. Cystic accumulation and abscess formation can occur at this level. The necrotic process follows the ischemic period. Necrotic areas will be walled with reactive fibrosis; necrotic areas extend with time and continued pressure to a coalescence and ultimately frank ulceration to the exterior. The process can extend deeper as well, causing superficially inapparent abscesses. Even frank ulcerations that appear superficially limited may have extensive tracking with second abscess activities underlying them. When abscesses extend to large fascial planes, extensive tracking occurs, as is the case when the psoas margin is involved, thus leading to a psoas abscess.

When extensive decubiti go through muscle, ultimate communication with bone is achieved that results in osteomyelitis. Persistent fever and elevated sedimentation rate in a patient with known decubitus ulcer should make the clinician suspect this entity. Deep abscess can of course also present with this picture. However, in the latter situation, films of the local bones and, if necessary, CT scan of the area should be done.

Computed tomography particularly has been shown to be of great help in the diagnosis of both deep abscess and osteomyelitis. This should also be done prior to any surgical procedure such as flap placement, in order to assess the extent of the decubital process accurately. Ulcers may also form over areas of heterotopic calcification.

It has been said that a decubitus ulcer is too often a sign of deficient medical care. There is no doubt that the prevention of decubitus formation has immeasurable benefit for both the patient and the medical personnel. As the pathophysiology of decubiti has come to be better and better understood, techniques have evolved that have paralleled this increased understanding.

Prevention of decubitus formation can be broken down into several large categories:

Turning

The immobilized patient must be turned from side to side every two hours *day and night.* In contradistinction to the normal person who shifts his position frequently even during sleep, presumably in response to noxious sensor stimuli emanating from pressure, the quadriplegic is doubly impaired. He can sense neither pressure nor pain, nor is he free to move spontaneously in even a random fashion.

The turning should be from side to side; in this way excessive sacral pressure is avoided. There are, however, other areas of the body that are subject to pressure forces. These include the ischial tuberosities, the heels, the spinous processes, the back of the head, and the trochanteric areas.

Pressure necrosis of the ischial tuberosities results from prolonged sitting. Care partners or attendants must be instructed in frequent lifting and repositioning of the patient to relieve ischial pressure.

Heel ulcerations are most commonly seen in the setting of a rough bedding surface and improperly fitting splint or shoes. Pressure to these areas can be prevented by the use of padded heel guards.

When spinal cord injury is combined with kyphotic deformity, pressure can result during prolonged sitting in a wheelchair. Thus, ulceration may occur at the site of the spinous processes. This can be prevented by attention to the padding on the back of seating surfaces.

Pressure necrosis of the back of the scalp can occur as a result of prolonged cervical traction. Therefore, frequent head repositioning is recommended in this situation. A full side-to-side turn is not necessary, but gentle change of position of even a few degrees (with adequate bolstering) is sufficient.

Although it is good practice to turn the patient from side to side frequently, side position can result in pressure on the trochanteric areas, with consequent breakdown. If a trochanteric breakdown occurs, turning must be alternated to prone-supine or uninvolved side positioning every two hours.

Surfaces

Special attention must be paid to the sleeping surface of the spinal cord injury patient. The use of egg crate mattresses, sheepskin, water and gel beds, and pneumatic mattresses all have been described. The use of specialized beds is not required in every case, since most standard beds can be adapted to the patient's individual needs.

In the evaluation of any positioning system, the degree of pressure and distribution should all be considered.

The same analysis of contact surfaces should obviously also be done for the patient's wheelchair. There are literally hundreds of seating surface adaptations available. It must be remembered, however, that any pressure more than 30 mm Hg may ultimately result in ulceration. Therefore, any common surface adaptation is never a substitute for adequate turning.

General Conditions

As will be elaborated upon in the chapter on nutrition, routine determinations of serum total protein and albumin levels are indicated in the evaluation of the quadriplegic patient. In general, it has been found that the patients whose serum albumin levels are below normal have a much greater likelihood of developing decubitus ulcers. Therefore, adequate nutrition and prevention or treatment of anemia are essential in the prevention (and, if necessary, the treatment) of pressure-related sores.

Associated medical illnesses, asthenic habitus, and prolonged bed rest are other important risk factors. Therefore, obviously, associated illnesses should be treated vigorously, and prolonged bed rest should be avoided in an attempt to forestall pressure related complications.

TREATMENT

When, despite the efforts enumerated above, a decubitus ulcer does occur, there are several large treatment concepts that must be kept in mind.

Superficial Excoriations

These can be treated conservatively with positioning (as mentioned above) and topical agents. These topicals include antibacterial agents and skin-soothing medications (such as Desitin® and Maalox®). Protective dressings may or may not be required in addition to topical medications.

Open Lesions

These may be of significant size but still remain within the connective tissue. Various dressings can be applied, and antiseptic materials (such as Betadine® or Daken's solution) have also been used. It should be noted that the use of caustic solutions, although helpful in cleaning the wound, may inhibit tissue granulation. Therefore, when the granulation phase begins, a switch should be made to noncaustic materials such as antibiotic ointments or saline dressings.

Porous, synthetic membrane-type dressings are also effective in the treatment of superficial lesions.

Deep Lesions

These are lesions that extend to deep connective tissue and superficial musculature. They are usually treated with hydrophyllic resins that enhance debridement. Surgical debridement can also be done at the bedside. Packing is also used to enhance healing by secondary intention.

It must be remembered that there will be no healing in the face of necrotic tissue. Debridement therefore is necessary to facilitate healing.

Lesions Penetrating to Bone and Deep Musculature

In the evaluation of deep lesions, and if there is suspicion of extension to bone, osteomyelitis must be expected and workup for this entity must be pursued aggressively. Some deep lesions can heal by secondary intention over prolonged periods of time, but surgical resolution may be required in many cases. The basis of surgical treatment in this condition is not aimed at approximation but rather at the use of split thickness skin grafts, myocutaneous flaps, and sometimes including surgical shaving of bony prominences. Before the patient is ready for any surgical procedure, however, the wound must be treated so that all necrotic tissue has been removed.

There are situations where even meticulous care does not prevent formation of pressure sores. Debilitated (and otherwise medically ill) patients with multiple decubiti ultimately have a higher risk of incurring amyloid disease. As a matter of fact, amyloid in quadriplegics has never been reported in the absence of decubitus disease. Unexplained liver or spleen enlargement, proteinuria, and unexplained elevated sedimentation rate all should bring up the question of amyloid. Gingival or rectal biopsy are usually diagnostic. The appearance of amyloidosis is a poor prognostic sign and is frequently associated with the terminal state in spinal cord injury patients.

SEBORRHEIC DERMATITIS

Quadriplegics have a higher than average incidence of seborrheic dermatitis. The reason for this is still unknown. The rash can be recognized as areas of erythema with scaly desquamation that may affect a major portion of the body surface area. The therapy for this condition is the administration of topical steroids, with the minimum dosage applied to the mucocutaneous junctions.

ACNE FLARE

Flare of acne vulgaris has a significant incidence in quadriplegia. This is due at least in part to the high incidence of quadriplegia in adolescents. In addition, the frequent use of high-dose systemic steroids as well as the presence of environmental stress contribute to this phenomenon. Treatment consists of meticulous skin care, avoidance of excess intake of sweets, and therapy with various medications. The latter include a variety of skin desquamative medications such as benzoyl peroxide. Recently, the use of vitamin A analogues in acne has also been described.

ALOPECIA AREATA

Alopecia areata is usually seen after significant and prolonged pressure on hair-bearing areas. This is seen with prolonged immobilization such as cervical traction, or after prolonged surgical procedures. It can be avoided by frequent turning.

TELOGEN EFFLUVIUM

Clinicians have often observed unusual cephalic hair loss in an even distribution beginning six to eight weeks after spinal cord injury. However, there is little in the literature to account for the etiology of this phenomenon. There has been some speculation that this hair loss may be due to episodes of fever. However, the pattern of hair loss in fever is usually typified by frontal and vertical thinning. In spinal cord injury patients, on the other hand, the pattern of hair loss is evenly dispersed.

Telogen effluvium has been described in association with various drug therapies, in schizophrenia, and also in overwhelming anxiety. It has also been reported in spinal cord injury,[3] and stress has been thought to be the cause of the factor in the patient under discussion. Whatever the cause, frequent clinical observations have been made of diffuse hair loss in spinal cord injury patients, which could be separated from the type of localized hair loss seen in malpositioning. Telogen effluvium is usually marked by prolonged hair loss over a period as long as one year, but in many patients, recovery and regrowth may be seen over a period of three to six months.

FUNGAL INFECTIONS

Fungal infections of the skin are frequent, annoying, and difficult to treat. The absence of spontaneous movement of areas of the body in quadriplegia engenders the persistence of warm, moist surfaces that are poorly ventilated. This makes the areas of skin susceptible to fungal infection. Therapy includes (1) frequent turning, (2) exposure of all surfaces (especially folds) to air, (3) good skin hygiene, especially in the setting of fecal or bladder incontinence. The use of antifungal creams, specifically either Lotrimin® or Mycostatin®, in addition to the above measures also has been helpful. The use of parenteral fungicides is usually not necessary, and griseofulvin, because of its side effects, is no longer recommended.

REFERENCES

1. Parsons K., Stawiski M.: Dermatologic complications of spinal cord injury. Annual meeting of ASCA, April 11–13, 1983.
2. Blumenthal F.A., et al.: A protective device for a decubitus ulcer. *A.P.M.R.* October 1970, pp. 611–613.
3. Cull J.G., et al.: A preliminary note on demographic and personality correlates of decubitus ulcer incidence. *J. Psychology* 85:225–227, 1973.
4. Burkhardt R.B.: An alternative to the total thigh flap for coverage of massive decubitus ulcers. *Plast. Reconstr. Surg.* 49:443–437, 1972.
5. Dietrick R.B., et al.: Tabulation and review of autopsy findings in fifty-five paraplegics. *J.A.M.A.* 166:41–44, 1958.
6. Edberg E.L., et al.: Prevention and treatment of pressure sores. *Phys. Ther.* 53:246–252, 1973.
7. Ferguson-Fell M.W., Wilkie I.C., Resnick J.B., et al.: Pressure sore prevention for the wheelchair-bound spinal cord injury patient. *Paraplegia* 18:42–51, 1980.
8. Hassard G.H.: Heterotopic bone formation about the hip and unilateral decubitus ulcers in spinal cord injury. *A.P.M.R.* 56:355–358, 1975.
9. Rogers E.C.: Nursing management in relation to beds used within the National Spinal Injuries Centre for the prevention of pressure sores. *Paraplegia* 16:147–153, 1978.
10. Putnam T., et al.: Sinography in management of decubitus ulcers. *A.P.M.R.* 59:243–245, 1978.
11. Richardson R.R., Meyer P.R.: Prevalence and incidence of pressure sores in acute spinal cord injuries. *Paraplegia* 19:235–247, 1982.
12. Shea J.: Pressure sores: Classification and management. *Clin. Orthop. Related Res.* 112:89–100, 1975.
13. Smith T.K., et al.: Complications associated with the use of the circular electrical turning frame. *J. Bone Joint Surg.* 57-A:711–713, 1975.
14. Stover S.L., et al.: Dermal fibrosis in spinal cord injury patients. *Arthritis Rheum.* 23:1312–1316, 1980.
15. Temes W.C., Harder P.: Pressure relief training device. *Phys. Ther.* 57:1152–1153, 1977.

12

Circulatory Complications

POSTURAL HYPOTENSION, autonomic crisis, and reflex bradycardia are all major circulatory complications of the quadriplegic state.

An understanding of the disordered physiology coupled with understanding of newer methods of prevention and therapy is essential if one is to successfully treat both acute and chronic cardiovascular manifestations in these patients.

AUTONOMIC CRISIS

Autonomic crisis is characterized by severe hypertension and bradycardia as well as by diaphoresis, headache, nasal congestion, agitation, chest pain, and miosis. This is usually seen in spinal cord injury above the level of T-6; it is occasionally seen in lesions of T-6 to T-8, but it is never seen in lesions below the level of T-10. Eighty percent of quadriplegics are said to have had this complication at one time or another. This constellation of symptoms is caused by massive sympathetic outflow in response to afferent stimulation below the level of the spinal cord lesion. This is seen in patients who have spinal cord transsection involving the lateral spinothalamic tract and the dorsal columns. In this situation, the sympathetic reflex arc (usually under the ultimate control of the hypothalamus) is deprived of its inhibitory input. Therefore, it can be said that although the sympathetics are present, their function is altered in high spinal cord lesions. Strong afferent input entering the cord below the site of the lesion thus causes facilitated and (unchecked) sympathetic activity. This in turn causes significant arterial constriction leading to severe hypertension. In response to the sudden and severe hypertension, reflex peripheral vasodilatation takes place with consequent flushing, sweating, and piloerection. Bradycardia is a result of the significant hypertension and is caused by stimulation of the vagus, especially at the carotid sinus. The most common afferent stimulus in quadriplegia arises from the distention of a hollow viscus. Bladder and bowel distention are the most common events culminating in autonomic dysfunction, although decubiti and decubital abscesses have also been implicated in the causation of this symptom complex.

In the rare situation where quadriplegia occurs in a pregnant woman, autonomic crisis has also been seen.[2]

Because the sympathetic preganglionic fibers are derived from levels T-1 to L-2 in the spinal cord, it is obvious that innervation for sweating does not correlate with the sensory dermatomes. The head, neck, and upper extremities are supplied by T-1 to 7, the trunk is supplied by T-4 to 12, and the lower extremities by T-9 to L-2. With interruption of the spinal cord above T-1, the sympathetic preganglionic fibers affecting sweating are deprived of hypothalamic control. Excessive sweating usually is not a clinical problem in itself. However, its association with the other signs of autonomic crisis makes it a good clinical indicator in the diagnosis of this entity.

When faced with the previously described clinical picture suggestive of autonomic crisis, the following steps should be undertaken:

1. A careful clinical examination in search of, for example, decubitus abscess or hollow viscus distention should be performed.
2. Under any circumstances, even without obvious bladder distention, urinary retention should be ruled out by straight catheterization.
3. If the patient is not found to be in urinary retention, evaluation for fecal impaction should be undertaken.

If these measures do not turn up a reversible cause for crisis, then pharmacologic therapy should be initiated.

Since postganglionic sympathetic fibers are cholinergic, Pro-Banthine® and Ditropan® (anticholinergic drugs) have been used with success in this entity. Mecomylamine (Inversine®), a ganglionic blocker, has also been used with good effect. Antihypertensive medications have had no effect on these symptoms.

If the syndrome of autonomic crisis goes untreated (or is treated inadequately) cerebral hemorrhage,[1] seizures, retinal hemorrhages, and occasionally death have been reported. In view of the severity of the symptoms and the serious complications of the phenomenon, it is doubly important to prevent even the onset of the syndrome. Patients with chronically high bladder residual volumes, chronically constipated persons, or patients with complicated decubiti are at risk and should be treated with the aforementioned medications on a prophylactic basis.

There are other situations where autonomic crisis has been reported. Manipulation of the urinary tract during genitourinary workup and the intraoperative state also have been responsible for hypertensive crisis. Spinal or epidural anesthesia in association with surgical procedures has been found to be helpful in preventing crisis.[1,3] Also, the use of ganglionic blockers (hexamethonium, guanethidine, trimethaphan, and pentolinium) have been effective in the treatment of autonomic crisis. Sympatholytic agents have not been useful in treatment.

Increase in prostaglandin E_2 may contribute to severe headache during hypertensive episodes.[29] This implies that aspirin, indomethacin and other prostaglandin inhibitors may be useful in relieving the headache associated with autonomic dysreflexia.

Many of the usual cardiac and vascular reflexes are altered in the quadriplegic. In these patients, resting blood pressures are usually lower than average. There is decreased myocardial contractility due to loss of sympathetic reflexes as well as an increase in venous capacitance. With increased venous capacitance, there is increased peripheral venous pooling as well as decreased venous return which in turn result in decreased cardiac output. All these factors contribute to the decrease of the cardiac reserve of the quadriplegic. In the normal individual, the Valsalva maneuver results in an increase in blood pressure secondary to increased intrathoracic pressure and in slowing of the heart rate secondary to vagus stimulation. In the quadriplegic, this maneuver results in a decrease in blood pressure and an increase in heart rate.[6]

The above factors of course have to be kept in mind when anesthesia is administered to patients with a high spinal cord injury.

For the patient with recent spinal cord injury, reflex bradycardia and even cardiac arrest can occur in response to endotracheal intubation or tracheal suctioning, especially in the face of hypoxia. In the patient with chronic spinal cord injury, this initial bradycardia is usually followed by severe blood pressure elevation as a response to visceral afferent stimuli. Under normal circumstances, endotracheal intubation causes high blood pressure and tachycardia. In the quadriplegic the bradycardia is likely caused by vasovagal reflex. Whereas reflexes are increased in the normal subject by sympathetic activity, this is obviously not the case in the quadriplegic. Because of this imbalance between parasympathetic and sympathetic stimuli leading to life-threatening bradycardia, it is suggested that quadriplegics undergoing intubation be pretreated with atropine. As stated previously, increased venous capacitance and decreased myocardial contractility are expected in patients with acute spinal cord lesions at or above the level of T-6.

Both factors contribute to the high incidence of pulmonary edema in these patients while undergoing anesthesia. Intravascular volume may be misjudged in quadriplegics because of the peripheral pooling of fluid. Therefore excess fluid may be given, a factor that is also frequently responsible for circulatory overload.

GENERAL ANESTHESIA

In the spinal cord injury patient, general anesthesia, with its well-known propensity for depression of myocardial function, is yet another etiologic factor for accidental circulatory overload. The use of arterial blood pressure lines and the Swan-

Ganz catheter (which measures pulmonary wedge pressure), central venous pressure lines, and frequent measurement of cardiac output by thermodilution studies all serve to give a much more accurate representation of the true state of circulating blood volume and biventricular function.

In patients with chronic spinal cord injury, especially those undergoing bladder surgery, intraoperative hypertensive crisis becomes a problem. To obviate this, halothane can be used as an anesthetic agent. Halothane acts either as a ganglionic blocker or as a suppressor of myocardial contractility, which in turn leads to a decrease in blood pressure. Spinal or epidural anesthesia is also effective because of its attendant ganglionic blocking effects. The most common ganglionic blocking agents used for prophylaxis and control of hypertensive crisis are hexamethonium, trimethaphan, and pentolinium. Succinylcholine should not be used as a ganglionic blocker because of the reported incidence of hyperkalemia after administration of the drug in patients with impaired neural function. Cardiovascular collapse evidently secondary to the hyperkalemia occurs in these patients after administration of this drug.

POSTURAL HYPOTENSION

Orthostatic hypotension is a major day-to-day problem in quadriplegics. Because of significant venous pooling as well as deficient vasomotor reflexes, there is a considerable decrease in blood pressure between the reclining and upright positions.

Blood pressure may diminish by as much as 30% to 50% in upright tilting. The heart rate may increase with the same maneuver.[4] In the early stages, the blood pressure drop may be so severe as to cause loss of consciousness. Of interest is the fact that systolic as well as diastolic blood pressure is decreased.

In the normal person, the change from the horizontal to the vertical position is accomplished without incident because of vasomotor reflexes that are responsible for maintenance of normal blood pressure in response to the gravity stimulus. In these normal persons the heart rate increases in response to the initial decrease in stroke volume. Thus, a combination of increased splanchnic return and increase in the heart rate compensate for the physiologic tendency to drop the blood pressure with orthostasis.

In response to the assumption of the vertical position from the horizontal, the quadriplegic experiences a drop in blood pressure with a rise in heart rate. The paralyzed muscles below the site of the spinal cord injury have decreased vascular tone, and thus there is an inability to respond in the usual way to the effects of gravity. The result is excessive venous pooling in the splanchnic inflow and in the extremities. The result of a decrease in venous return thus causes hypotension. Tachycardia, which in a normal individual is only one of the compensatory mechanisms, is also seen. This is the only intact compensatory mechanism in the quadriplegic. This is not sufficient to increase blood pressure in the upright position, however. Thus, the quadriplegic has hypotension and tachycardia with the attendant ultimate symptoms of decreased cerebral blood flow.

As far as the sympathetic response to tilting is concerned, serum dopamine β-hydroxylase and plasma renin activities have been found to increase significantly 15 minutes after tilt. This suggests that reflex sympathetic stimulation persists despite cervical cord transsection. Other possibilities for an intact renin response have been suggested. These include (1) reflex sympathetic activity in the isolated spinal cord and (2) decrease in renal perfusion pressure leading to increased renin activity. Of interest also is the fact that levels of ADH, cortisol, and prostaglandin E_2 as well as norepinephrine also rise on tilting in the quadriplegic. As far as norepinephrine is concerned, there is an increase with tilt table in both normal persons and quadriplegics. However, there is a delay in the peak of norepinephrine production in quadriplegics.

Although there are far-reaching suppositions as far as the etiology of postural hypotension is concerned, the treatment had remained the same for many years. Most patients undergoing gradual tilt table positioning ultimately develop tolerance of the vertical position. Therefore this is really the most important therapeutic modality for this condition. Tilt table can be discontinued when the patient is able to tolerate the sitting position without untoward symptoms. The mechanism for this acquired response is not clear.

In combination with the tilting exercises, abdominal binders should be used during upright hours. The effect of the binder is to decrease venous pooling in the visceroabdominal vasculature. Although inflatable leg cuffs, elastic stockings, and other means of promoting venous return from the lower extremities have been used, studies have shown that abdominal pressure is more effective in achieving this goal.[5] Inflatable air pads can be placed within the abdominal binder in order to increase abdominal pressure further.

Biofeedback[4] has also been used for the treatment of postural hypotension, but the number of cases in this study was small.

CONCLUSION

Postural hypotension early in the course of quadriplegia is almost universal. The outlook for complete tolerance to the upright position is excellent, with the combination of tilt table exercises and means described for promoting increased venous return.

REFERENCES

1. Neider R.M., et al.: Autonomic hyperreflexia in urologic surgery. *J.A.M.A.* 213:867–869, 1970.
2. Nath M., et al.: Autonomic hyperreflexia in pregnancy and labor: A case report. *Am. J. Obstet. Gynecol.* 134:390–392, 1979.
3. Muravchick S., et al.: Pentolinium for control of reflex hypertension in spinal cord injured patients. *Paraplegia* 16:350–356, 1978.
4. Huang C.-T., et al.: Cardiopulmonary response in spinal cord injury patients: Effect of pneumatic compressive devices. *A.P.M.R.* 64:101–106, 1983.
5. Bruckner B.S.: Biofeedback as an experimental treatment for postural hypotension in a patient with a spinal cord lesion. *A.P.M.R.* 58:49–53, 1977.
6. Welpy N.C., Mathias C.J., Frankel H.L.: Circulation reflexes in tetraplegics during artificial ventilation and general anesthesia. *Paraplegia* 13:172–182, 1975.
7. Bake B., et al.: Breathing patterns and regional ventilation distribution in tetraplegic patients and in normal subjects. *Clin. Sci.* 42:117–126, 1972.

8. Claus-Walker J., et al.: Hypertensive episodes in quadriplegic patients: Neuro-endocrine mechanisms.
9. Eidelberg E.E.: Cardiovascular response to experimental spinal cord compression. *J. Neurosurg.* 38:326–331, 1973.
10. Fast A.: Reflex sweating in patients with spinal cord injury: A review. *A.P.M.R.* 58:435–437, 1977.
11. Frankel H.L., et al.: Severe hypertension in patients with high spinal cord lesions undergoing electro-ejaculation—management with prostaglandin E_2. *Paraplegia* 18:293–299, 1980.
12. Fugl-Meyer A.R., Grimby G.: Rib-cage and abdominal volume ventilation partitioning in tetraplegic patients. *Scand. J. Rehabil. Med.* 3:161–167, 1971.
13. Kamelhar D.L., et al.: Plasma renin and serum dopamine-β-hydroxylase during orthostatic hypotension in quadriplegic man. *A.P.M.R.* 59:212–216, 1978.
14. Keltz H., et al.: Effect of quadriplegia and hemidiaphragmatic paralysis on thoraco-abdominal pressure during respiration. *Am. J. Phys. Med.* 48:109–115, 1969.
15. Mathias C.J., et al.: Dopamine β-hydroxylase release during hypertension from sympathetic nervous overactivity in man. *Cardiovasc. Res.* 10:176–181, 1976.
16. Mathias C.J., et al.: Plasma catecholamines during paroxysmal neurogenic hypertension in quadriplegic man. *Circ. Res.* 39:204–208, 1976
17. McCluer S.: A temporary method of controlling orthostatic hypotension in quadriplegia. *Prosth. Orthop. Devices* (submitted Jan. 22, 1968) pp. 598–599.
18. Nanninga J.B., et al.: Effect of autonomic hyperreflexia on plasma renin. *Urology* 7:638–640, 1976.
19. Senter H.J., et al.: Altered blood flow and secondary injury in experimental spinal cord trauma. *J. Neurosurg.* 49:569–578, 1978.
20. Senter H.J., et al.: Loss of autoregulation and post-traumatic ischemia following experimental spinal cord trauma. *J. Neurosurg.* 50:198–206, 1979.
21. Senter H.J., et al.: Alteration of posttraumatic ischemia in experimental spinal cord trauma by a central nervous system depressant. *J. Neurosurg.* 50:207–216, 1979.
22. Shoenfeld Y., et al.: Orthostatic hypotension in amputees and subjects with spinal cord injuries. *A.P.M.R.* 59:138–141, 1978.
23. Snow J.C., et al.: Cardiovascular collapse following succinylcholine in a paraplegic patient. *Paraplegia* 11:199–204, 1973.

24. Gabriele F.T.: Anesthesia of the spinal cord injured patient: cardiovascular problems and their management. *Paraplegia* 13: 162–171, 1975.
25. Vallbona C., et al.: Control of orthostatic hypotension of quadriplegic patients with a pressure suit. *A.P.M.R.* 44:7–18, 1963.
26. Walters J.M., Nott M.R.: The hazards of anesthesia in the injured patient. *Br. J. Anaesth.* 49:707–720, 1977.
27. Naftchi N.E., et al.: Hypertensive crises in quadriplegic patients: Changes in cardiac output, blood volume, serum dopamine-β-hydroxylase activity, and arterial prostaglandin PGE_2. *Circulation* 57:336–341, 1978.
28. Naftchi N.E., et al.: Relationship between serum dopamine-β-hydroxylase activity, catecholamine metabolism, and hemodynamic changes during paroxysmal hypertension in quadriplegia. *Circ. Res.* 35:850–861, 1974.
29. Berk J.L., Levy M.N.: Profound reflex bradycardia produced by transient hypoxia or hypercapnia in man. *Eur. Surg. Res.* 9:75–84, 1977.
30. Corbett J.L., et al.: Cardiovascular responses to tilting in tetraplegic man. *J. Physiol.* 215:411–431, 1971.
31. Fluck D.C., et al.: Effect of tilting on plasma catecholamine levels in man. *Cardiovasc. Res.* 7:823–826, 1973.
32. Ibrahim M.M., et al.: Orthostatic hypotension: Mechanisms and management. *Am. Heart J.* 90:513–520, 1975.
33. Johnson R.H., Park D.M.: Effect of change of posture on blood pressure and plasma renin concentration in men with spinal transections. *Clin. Sci.* 44:539–546, 1973.
34. Love D.R., et al.: Plasma renin in idiopathic orthostatic hypotension: Differential response in subjects with probable afferent and efferent autonomic failure. *Clin. Sci.* 41:239–299, 1971.
35. Mendelsohn F.A., Johnston C.I.: Renin release in chronic paraplegia. *Aust. Nzj. Med.* 4:393–397, 1971.
36. Polinsky R.J., et al.: Sympathetic prosthesis for managing orthostatic hypotension. *Lancet* 901–904, 1983.
37. Schonwald G.: Cardiovascular complications during anesthesia in chronic spinal cord injured patients. *Anesthesiology* 55:550–558, 1981.
38. Vallbona C.: Endocrine responses to orthostatic hypotension in quadriplegia. *Arch. Phys. Med. Rehabil.* 47:412–421, 1966.

13

Endocrine Complications

IT HAS BEEN SHOWN that spinal cord injury can cause systemic effects removed from the actual anatomic site of trauma. Endocrine changes have been found often in incidental fashion during systemic testing in these patients. This in turn has led to further research into the hormonal abnormalities associated with spinal cord injury.

In general, significant clinical acumen is required to make a diagnosis of endocrinopathy in all but the most flagrant manifestations of endocrine disease. In the quadriplegic who frequently exhibits a host of potentially confusing symptoms and, frequently, an absence of characteristic physical findings, endocrine disorders are even more difficult to diagnose. Thus it is of the utmost importance to be alert to the presence of hormone-related abnormalities that may subtly impede progress or complicate another, already existing, medical illness.

HYPERCALCEMIA

It is quite common for immobilized patients to have hypercalciuria and osteoporosis. Hypercalciuria begins in the acute postinjury period. Definite osteoporosis is evident within the first six months after injury. The sequelae of hypercalciuria are discussed in the genitourinary chapter. Osteoporosis has been discussed in the musculoskeletal chapter.

Immobilization hypercalcemia is a relatively rare complication of immobilization due to spinal cord injury. It is almost invariably seen in the male adolescent population and is seen within four to eight weeks after injury. Young spinal-cord-injured men are immobilized after many years of energetic physical activity. During this time, bone formation and resorption are essentially in balance. At the time of immobilization, however, bone formation is decreased while the rate of resorption remains elevated. The kidneys of patients in whom hypercalcemia does develop cannot adequately clear calcium derived from trabecular bone. The exact mechanism for this has not been elucidated.

Adrenocortical insufficiency has been mentioned as a possible contributing cause to immobilization hypercalcemia. It is well known that hypercalcemia occurs in adrenal insufficiency. In the patient reported by Steinberg et al.,[5] decreased adrenal function values and elevated levels of ACTH were seen in an immobilized patient with hypercalcemia. Steroid administration diminished the serum calcium level in this patient. On the other hand, steroids diminish calcium in multiple hypercalcemic states, so that one need not necessarily postulate adrenal insufficiency as an explanation for the calcium lowering effect of steroids.

As is the case in hypercalcemia in non–spinal-cord-injured persons, this entity may present with a bewildering constellation of symptoms. The major symptoms include anorexia, nausea, obstipation, and headache. Polydipsia and polyuria, listlessness, and ultimately seizures and coma are other symptoms that should alert the clinician to the presence of this entity. The major symptoms may easily be overlooked and misinterpreted as nonspecific complaints of the spinal-cord-injured patient. It is therefore highly important to consider the diagnosis of hypercalcemia early, so that proper therapy can be instituted before a life-threatening situation occurs.

The diagnosis of immobilization hypercalcemia, therefore, is based on the presence of hypercalcemia and hypercalciuria, usually in a previously physically active adolescent male. The level of parathyroid hormone is normal; of interest is the fact that the alkaline phosphatase level is normal as well. The reason for the latter is that, in this condition, there is a significant diminution of osteoblastic activity, thus lowering the usually elevated alkaline phosphatase level of adolescence to normal.

Therapy of Hypercalcemia

Once the diagnosis of immobilization hypercalcemia has been made, the hypercalcemia should be treated very much in the same way as hypercalcemia of other etiologies in non–spinal-cord-injured persons.

Therapy is aimed at the rapid lowering of serum calcium. This is best accomplished by the administration of sodium chloride. Calcium is excreted in parallel with sodium, and therefore the vigorous administration of sodium chloride with consequently increased sodium excretion is associated with an increased excretion of calcium. The concurrent administration of furosemide or ethacrynic acid promotes calciuria with consequent lowering of serum calcium secondary to decreased sodium and calcium tubular reabsorption.

It is the unusual case in which one has to resort to additional agents for the therapy of hypercalcemia. Phosphates, which can be given either by mouth (such as by the administration of Fleet's Phospho-soda) or $Na_2H_3PO_4$ given intravenously, have a significant serum calcium lowering effect. Corticosteroids have been used for many years for the treatment of hypercalcemia. As was discussed previously, steroids do lower the calcium level in patients with adrenal insufficiency. However, by far the largest incidence of the use of corticosteroids is in hypercalcemia with normal adrenal function.

In summary, most patients with immobilization hypercalcemia respond to hydration with or without the use of furosemide or ethacrynic acid. Most of the patients who do not respond to these modalities will likely respond to the administration of phosphate or ultimately to the administration of corticosteroids. It must be emphasized, however, that the above therapeutic modalities are useful primarily for the acute hypercalcemic state.

Early remobilization of the spinal cord injury patient may

well prevent the occurrence of hypercalcemia. Once it has occurred, however, early weight bearing and tilt table should be instituted concomitant with the therapy of hypercalcemia. This effect of early weight bearing is drawn from NASA studies of bone formation and resorption during periods of weightlessness. However, in other studies[4,6] it was found that immobilization hypercalcemia can occur even in persons who are passively weight bearing (e.g., sitting in a chair). This implies that both weight bearing and mobilization (ranging) are necessary for the treatment or prevention of this disorder.

THYROID DYSFUNCTION

It is difficult to assess the true incidence of hypothyroidism in *association* with quadriplegia. In one study[1] there was an incidence of 0.9% of hypothyroidism in a spinal-cord-injured population. In view of the difficulty in assessing the true incidence of hypothyroidism in the population at large (the number of undiagnosed hypothyroids is presumably significant), it is difficult to compare this incidence with that of the general population. Although low serum T_4 levels have been observed in acute quadriplegia,[2] a more recent study[1] did not show any abnormalities of T_4 levels in spinal cord injured patients as compared with normal controls. Certainly a low serum T_4 level should alert the clinician to the possible presence of hypothyroidism. However, since there can be other causes of a low T_4 (thyroid binding globulin (TBG) deficiency, administration of androgen or diphenylhydantoin) a thyroid stimulating hormone (TSH) sample should be drawn before therapy is started. An elevated level of thyroid-stimulating hormone together with a borderline or low T_4 level is certainly suggestive of hypothyroidism. Before any thyroid therapy is started, however, assessment of pituitary and adrenal function should also be carried out in order to rule out concomitant or causative abnormalities in other endocrine organs.

All in all, the incidence of hypothyroidism does not appear to be of major importance in the clinical evaluation of the spinal-cord-injured population, which is predominantly young and male.

As far as hyperthyroidism is concerned in these patients, there has been no extensive study that has dealt with hyperthyroidism solely in the spinal-cord-injured population.

GLUCOSE METABOLISM

Fasting blood sugar levels in patients with chronic spinal cord injury (duration more than eight months) have, in one study, been found to be in the low-normal range.[4] Glucose tolerance curves were found to be below normal in chronic spinal cord injury patients.[4] In spinal cord injured patients under stress (such as surgery), inappropriate increases of blood sugar were noted intraoperatively.

In another study[3] (albeit one with a small number of patients), it was found that 30% of spinal cord injury patients had a two-hour after-glucose load value of over 200 mg/ml. Forty percent of the patients had values exceeding 140 mg% under the same conditions. In a retrospective study of 57 discharged spinal cord injury patients, 23 had fasting hyperglycemia. These values of course exceed what one would expect in a predominantly male and under age 30 group without spinal cord injury.

The mechanism of the hyperglycemia in these patients appears to be that of endogenous insulin resistance. Exogenous insulin resistance was also demonstrated. There was no increase in the level of glucagon or growth hormone, and the endogenous insulin produced eluted in the same peak as authentic insulin.

Although no other endocrine cause for the hyperglycemia was found, it has been proposed that muscle wasting is somehow related to hyperinsulinemia, as has been postulated for the same abnormality in myotonic dystrophy.

GONADAL ABNORMALITIES

In males with spinal cord injury, there is a normal basal testosterone level, except in the acute period when this value is low. There is abnormal spermatogenesis both in the acute and chronic phase. This is thought to be secondary to abnormally high scrotal temperature due to interruption of lumbar sympathetic nerve supply, further complicated by absence of the cremasteric reflex. On testicular biopsy in these patients the morphological findings are usually normal, but spermatogenic arrest may be seen with hypoplasia of the germinal epithelium. Motile spermatozoa are markedly diminished in these patients. There have been reports of high as well as low 17-kerosteroid levels in quadriplegics.[7] Increased urinary estrogen levels have also been reported.[7] Gynecomastia has also been reported in male quadriplegics.[8]

As far as gonadotrophins are concerned, increased basal follicle stimulating hormone with exaggerated response of LRH to exposure to FSH has been reported in one third of 18 of the patients in one study.[7]

Very little has been written about menstrual abnormalities in women with spinal cord injury. Jeanne A. Epstein, M.D., in a personal communication (1983), stated that, in her clinical experience of six spinal-cord-injured women, these patients had normal menstrual function and the usual fertility potential of neurologically normal women of comparable age. She felt on the basis of these facts, that the hypothalamic-pituitary-ovarian axis is intact in these patients.

REFERENCES

1. Prakash V., Lin M.S., Chung H.A., et al.: Thyroid hypofunction in spinal cord injury patients. *Paraplegia* 18:56–63, 1980.
2. Claus-Walker J., Spencer W.A., Carter R.E., et al.: Bone metabolism in quadriplegia: Dissociation between calciuria and hydroxyprolinuria. *Arch. Phys. Med. Rehabil.* 56:327–332, 1975.
3. Duckworth C.C., Jallepalli P., Solomon S.S.: Glucose intolerance in spinal cord injury. *A.P.M.R.* 65:107–110, 1983.
4. Claus-Walker J.: Metabolic and endocrine changes in spinal cord injury: II. Partial decentralization of the autonomic nervous system. *A.P.M.R.* 63:569–575, 1982.
5. Steinberg F.U., Birge S.J., Cooke N.E.: Hypercalcaemia in adolescent tetraplegic patients: Case report and review. *Paraplegia* 16:60–67, 1978.
6. Maynard J.E., Melmed S.: Immobilization hypercalcemia in spinal cord injury. *Metabolism* 28:1051–1075, 1979.
7. Morley J.E., Melmed S.: Gonadal dysfunction in systemic disorders. *Metabolism* 28:1051, 1979.

8. Kikuchi T.A., Skowsky R.W., El Toraei I., et al.: The pituitary-gonadal axis in spinal cord injury. *Fertil. Steril.* 27:1142–1145, 1975.

9. Claus-Walker J.: Metabolic and endocrine changes in spinal cord injury: I. The nervous system before and after transection of the spinal cord. *A.P.M.R.* 62:595–601, 1981.

10. Hanson R.W., Franklin M.R.: Sexual loss in relation to other functional losses for spinal cord injured males. *A.P.M.R.* 57:291–293, 1976.

11. Naftchi N.E., Viau A.T., Sell G.H., et al.: Pituitary-gonadal axis dysfunction in spinal cord injury. *A.P.M.R.* 57:551, 555, 1976.

12. Vemireddi N.K.: Sexual counseling for chronically disabled patients. *Geriatrics,* July 1978, pp. 65–69.

13. Wortsman J., Burns G., Van Beck A.L., et al.: Hyperadrenergic state after trauma to the neuroaxis. *J.A.M.A.* 243:1459–1460, 1980.

14

Nutrition in the Quadriplegic Patient

IT MAY NOT BE immediately apparent that there are frequent and severe problems in nutrition in the quadriplegic patient. Many other clinical events overshadow this particular problem, so that one may be faced with an undernourished patient in a relatively acute way.

There are many reasons for undernourishment in the quadriplegic. These include, among the causes of diminished intake, degrees of loss of hand function (with resulting need for assistive devices or the help of another person for feeding), diminished appetite due to depression, and intercurrent medical problems requiring parenteral nutrition. On occasion, nasogastric tube placement may be necessary and may thus engender malnutrition if used for a long time and if parenteral hyperalimentation is not employed.

Less well known as causes of malnutrition in the quadriplegic are increased metabolic requirements of various causes. The causative factors of these increased requirements include such factors as the presence of decubitus ulcer, the repair of tissue after surgical procedures, and, of course, the catabolic consequences of the original injury.

To fully understand the nutritional requirements of quadriplegics, it is also necessary to encapsulate the major changes in fluid and electrolyte balance following spinal cord injury. The spinal cord injury patient has a higher extracellular volume (ECV) to intracellular volume (ICV) ratio, something that is especially marked during the acute phase after injury. There is a higher than normal exchangeable sodium level and a lower than normal exchangeable potassium level as compared to non–spinal-cord-injured persons. All of this has resulted in the inability of these persons to tolerate elevated levels of hydration.

Because of the higher ECV, these patients are at risk of fluid overload. Thus, all IV fluid flow rates must be monitored carefully. This is especially true in the administration of hypertonic solutions, such as in parenteral hyperalimentation. It is also noteworthy that, during hyperalimentation, the spinal cord injured patient experiences hypercalciuria, so that adequate amounts of calcium must be added to the hyperalimentation solution.[1] The use of parenteral calcium supplementation ensures that exogenous calcium will be lost in the urine, thus preventing the leaching of endogenous calcium from bone.

The appearance of bilateral lower extremity edema in these patients may be troubling to the physician. This finding, in the face of normal test results for deep venous obstruction, reflects the higher ECV and can be easily resolved through the use of compression garments, elevation, and ranging of the lower extremities. Sodium restriction and use of diuretics should not be used. The quadriplegic, especially during the acute postinjury phase, reacts poorly to sodium restriction, which can result in the diminution of an already diminished ICV, and this ultimately results in worsening of the already significant postural hypotension. If diuretics are also added, orthostatic problems may become even more severe.[2]

The spinal cord injured patient has a lower than average exchangeable potassium level, which in some cases may lead to a sensation of tightness in the lower extremities even in the absence of true pain.[3]

It should be stated that progressive muscular atrophy leads to further potassium depletion. It may therefore be necessary to replete the potassium of the spinal cord injured patient, preferably by dietary supplementation. According to Pfeiffer et al.,[4] there are certain definitive criteria for the identification of the patient who is at nutritional risk. These include (1) a body weight 10% below the ideal body weight; (2) calorie and protein intake that does not meet anabolic or at least maintenance requirements; (3) a serum albumin concentration less than 3 gm/dL; (4) a hemoglobin value below 12 gm and a hematocrit reading below 37%; and (5) a creatinine-height index (a reflection of muscle mass) of less than 60% of standard.

As far as body weight is concerned, weight loss is usually noted in the early stages of spinal cord injury. This is due to a combination of factors including atrophy of muscle, as well as diminished dietary intake. The latter is usually in association with loss of upper extremity function for feeding and prolonged maintenance on parenteral fluids without concomitant oral intake. During this period, the shift leading to a higher proportion of ECV vs. ICV begins. Lower body weight places the patient at greater nutritional risk as well as at greater risk for the development of decubitus ulcers.

By about six months after injury, a gradual weight gain may be noticed, which is then sustained in later years. This is explained by replacement of atrophied muscles by fat and increased facility with self-feeding. Decreased caloric requirements due to inactivity are outstripped by normal or excess caloric intake, also resulting in weight gain. It should again be emphasized that the serum albumin level is a rough but useful index of general nutritional status. A low albumin level frequently is associated with poor healing of decubiti and wounds in general.

There has been much controversy in the literature about the use of low-calcium diets in spinal cord injury. The supporters of the low-calcium diet have maintained that this regimen can prevent the formation of renal stones and the development of immobilization hypercalcemia. Although it has been the custom in some rehabilitation centers to keep patients calcium restricted, the recent trend in most centers seems to be in the direction of normal calcium diets. It is well known, however, that urinary tract stone formation in spinal cord injury patients is due rather to infections with urea-splitting organisms such as *Proteus* with concomitant alkalinization of the urine and consequent crystal formation than to hypercalciuria per se.[6] Therefore (as discussed elsewhere), maintenance of a patent urinary tract, adequate hydration, and treatment of urinary tract infections are the cornerstones of prevention of stone formation in these patients.

It must be kept in mind that males in the 14-to-23 age range are especially at risk for immobilization hypercalcemia.[5] As discussed in the endocrine chapter, the patients in this age group are already in a state of high metabolic turnover at the time of injury. With the higher bone turnover associated with the acute phase of spinal cord injury, added to the age-related metabolic flux, it can be understood that these patients may well be at risk for hypercalcemia.

Although the main body of data in this subject applies to males, it stands to reason that patients of both sexes should have careful attention paid to calcium metabolism.

Concomitantly, a spinal cord injured patient with nausea, vomiting, constipation, or polyuria (singly or in combination) should be suspected of having hypercalcemia. (A detailed discussion of the diagnosis and therapy of hypercalcemia can be found in the endocrine chapter.)

It should also be remembered that an across-the-board institutional low-calcium diet can in itself cause significant nutritional problems in the quadriplegic. A low-calcium diet is obviously restricted in dairy products, and therefore it is difficult to ensure an adequate protein intake in a population already at nutritional risk.

ANEMIA

Anemia is an ever-present problem in the spinal cord injury population, particularly in the immediate prostraumatic period. There have been multiple theories proposed for the etiology of this anemia. These include shifts in volume[7] causing dilutional changes, associated chronic disorder (such as decubitus ulcer), and infection.[7] Erythropoietin levels have been done in these situations but have shown variable results.[8] Although erythropoietin levels themselves have not been uniformly diminished, it has been postulated that there is decreased target cell sensitivity to erythropoietin in these patients, thus causing the anemia.

Whatever the etiology, anemia is a disturbing clinical factor in the quadriplegic. As is always the case, a thorough workup as far as red blood cell indices, RBC morphology, and indications of hemolysis is indicated. Obviously, chronic or acute bleeding should be ruled out. Uremia and occult infection should be searched for as well.

If, as is commonly the case, no obvious source is found, it is advisable to treat the patient expectantly, by keeping a careful eye on nutrition as well as on iron, vitamin, and folate requirements. Ultimately, in those patients in whom no obvious source for the anemia is found, the anemia resolves spontaneously within several months after trauma.

It should also be stated that the usual anemia (in other words, that without obvious cause) tends to be mild. If, for example, the anemia is so severe as to dictate the use of transfusion, it is more likely that an obvious source will be found.

CONCLUSION

In summary, it can be stated quite simply that adequate nutrition is one of the cornerstones of the prevention and treatment of many of the medical complications of quadriplegia. In the immediate post-trauma period, and even with the best of care, the concept of adequate nutrition may sometimes take a back seat to urgent considerations such as maintenance of respiration, treatment of abdominal trauma, and other acute medical and surgical problems. After the acute phase is over, maintenance of gastric intubation and consequent need for intravenous hydration as well as difficulties with self-feeding, depression, etc. all may subtly influence the initiation of a state of undernutrition. Catabolic causes such as decubitus ulcers and/or increased caloric requirements such as healing wounds all may contribute to this state.

Calcium, sodium, and potassium requirements are all in a

state of flux in the spinal cord injury patient and must be carefully monitored. Low-grade anemia is frequently seen in the spinal cord injury patient, and if no overt cause is found it is usually self-limited.

All in all, nutrition is an important and frequently underestimated variable in the care of the spinal cord injury patient.

REFERENCES

1. Claus-Walker J., et al.: Increased urine calcium during hyperalimentation in quadriplegia: Report of two cases. *A.P.M.R.* 62:347–349, 1981.
2. Claus-Walker J., et al.: Metabolic effects of sodium restriction and thiazides in tetraplegic patients. *Paraplegia* 15:3–10, 1977.
3. Claus-Walker J., et al.: Metabolic and endocrine changes in spinal cord injury: I. The nervous system before and after transection of the spinal cord. *A.P.M.R.* 62:595–601, 1981.
4. Pfeiffer S.C., et al.: Nutritional assessment of the spinal cord injured patient. *J. Am. Dietetic Assoc.* 78:501–504, 1981.
5. Claus-Walker J., et al.: Metabolic and endocrine changes in spinal cord injury: IV. Compounded neurologic dysfunction. *A.P.M.R.* 63:632–638, 1982.
6. Claus-Walker J., et al.: Electrolytes in urinary calculi and urine of patients with spinal cord injuries. *A.P.M.R.,* 54:109–114, 1973.
7. Perkash A., Brown M.: Anaemia in patients with traumatic spinal cord injury. *Paraplegia* 20:235–236, 1982.
8. Claus-Walker J., et al.: Spinal cord injury and serum erythropoietin. *A.P.M.R.,* 65:370–374, 1984.
9. Bildstein C., et al.: Nutritional management of a patient with brain damage and spinal cord injury. *A.P.M.R.,* 64:382–383, 1983.
10. Claus-Walker J., et al.: Metabolic and endocrine changes in spinal cord injury: II. Consequences of partial decentralization of the autonomic nervous system. *A.P.M.R.,* 63:569–575, 1982.
11. Claus-Walker J., et al.: Metabolic and endocrine changes in spinal cord injury: II. Partial decentralization of the autonomic nervous system. *A.P.M.R.,* 63:576–580, 1982.
12. Claus-Walker J., et al.: Metabolic and endocrine changes in spinal cord injury: III. Less quanta of sensory input plus bedrest and illness. *A.P.M.R.,* 63:628–631, 1982.
13. Claus-Walker J., et al.: Spinal cord injury hypercalcemia: Therapeutic profile. *A.P.M.R.,* 63:108–115, 1982.

15

Psychosexual Adjustment to Spinal Cord Injury

ANGELO R. CANEDO, PH.D.

THE AREA OF SEXUALITY and sexual behavior after spinal cord injury has engendered an increasing amount of research over the last two decades. This research is part of the overall increase in attention that has been paid to issues of human sexuality by both medical and behavioral scientists. The sum of this research supports the view that sexual adjustment is an integral factor in the individual's total psychological adjustment.[14]

There appears to be a strong correlation between the spinal cord injury patient's reports on sexual satisfaction and his or her overall satisfaction with life.[2, 21] This is noted to be the case for both paraplegic and quadriplegic persons.

The question of how an individual adjusts to a specific disability is a complex one and is more specifically addressed in the chapter on psychological adjustment to spinal cord injury. Overall adjustment to the disability is mitigated by a number of factors, including the individual's premorbid life-style and personality dynamics as well as by his social, cultural, economic, and familial concerns. Even the circumstances that led to the injury affect their reactions to the disability.

Recent studies indicate that sexual adjustment may play a

more critical role than was acknowledged previously. Some studies indicate that there is even a correlation between success in vocational rehabilitation and sexual adjustment.[6] It therefore appears that sexual behavior has many social and psychological ramifications and is not dictated purely by physiology.[10]

The maintenance of objectivity and the offering of candid, comprehensive professional advice are critical in sexual counseling. The therapist needs to be particularly careful in not subtly communicating discomfort with a particular issue. Sensitivity is crucial in allaying anxiety and discomfort on the part of the disabled person who is asking for help.

The patient may ask what seem to be simplistic questions, or he may not be able to formulate his questions in precise technical terms. The disabled individual may not be versed in the specific anatomy of the genitalia and thus may be unsure of how to ask for information. Embarrassment about asking questions often perpetuates this ignorance. The clinician needs to be sensitive, practical, and at ease with the topic. Providing specific information in understandable terms will help to decrease the patient's anxiety about discussing the topic and make it easier to ask more pertinent questions. Specific information about particular treatments, interventions, techniques, and behavior can be communicated easily and addressed openly if the clinician is skilled and sensitive to the patient's concerns.

The clinician's own psychosexual attitudes are a major factor to be considered in his sexual counseling of others. Medical and nursing personnel are frequently called on to provide sexual counseling to spinal cord injury patients. For these non-professional therapists it is extremely important that they be aware of their own sexual attitudes so that they do not inadvertently project their values on the spinal cord injury patient whose sexuality is often in flux.

In the final analysis the patient's behavior is based on what is comfortable for him. The physician can provide for the patient complete information on the ramifications of spinal cord injury along with information on sexual alternatives and options.

SEXUAL DESIRE AND SATISFACTION IN THE SPINAL CORD INJURED

Sexual desire and libido seem to remain unchanged in spinal cord injury patients. What seems to diminish in some cases is the feeling of sexual satisfaction.[21, 23] This may be due to a lack of education about the sexual aspects of their disabilities. Providing spinal cord injury patient's with information about the specifics of their sexuality seems to have a positive impact in many cases.[16] While some feel that the level of sexual satisfaction in the spinal cord injured may decrease from self-reported premorbid levels, most of these individuals still see sexuality as a satisfactory experience.[23] In fact, many studies indicate that the drive for sexual satisfaction is not negatively affected. Desire and interest seem to stay consistent with what would have been expected prior to injury.[5, 21, 24]

Sexuality issues do not seem to be of primary concern to most patients during the very early period post injury. Some may view this limited emphasis on sexuality while demonstrating greater concern over their ambulatory status (for example) as another facet of denial. An alternative view is that, as noted, sexuality becomes a more pronounced issue after the patient has dealt with the more basic issues and is ready to face a period of social reentry and acclimatization.

FEARS ABOUT SEXUALITY AFTER SPINAL CORD INJURY

Spinal-cord-injured persons may shy away from expressing their sexual desires because they feel inferior, undesirable, weak, helpless, or unable to perform as an equal with their prospective partner. Many spinal cord injury patients must deal with a number of major issues before overcoming their concerns about their sexuality. They must first deal with an impaired sense of body image often accompanied by decreased self-esteem leading to concerns about gender identity and role. There are also concerns about the ability to participate and to offer something positive in terms of a couples relationship and later in terms of a parent figure. Lastly, they may also have concerns about their sexual capabilities as a partner.[27]

Fears of intimacy may therefore be related to premorbid concerns, to changes in body image, to fears of rejection on a number of issues, or to feelings of low self-esteem and worthlessness. While there is much less research to date on the sexual adjustment concerns of spinal-cord-injured women compared with men, it seems that many of the initial reactions and concerns are similar. However, along with the more social aspects discussed previously, both sexes seem to show some initial concern about fertility. Men are concerned with issues of sexual potency, while women often worry about their ability to conceive and their capacity to carry a pregnancy to term.

For both men and women there are usually some concerns about more practical problems such as the fear of having a bowel or bladder accident during sexual activity. There is an understandable although often almost extreme preoccupation with avoiding such embarrassment. In addition, there frequently are concerns about whether there are any other sanitary or health implications. There are concerns about positioning, worries about spasticity, body temperature changes, and a host of other physical concerns that need to be clarified so as to avoid panic reactions that then might lead to an avoidance of sexual encounters.

In short, persons with spinal cord injuries need to be educated at first and then encouraged to develop positive and realistic attitudes about themselves as sexual beings.

THE CONCERNS OF PARTNERS AND SIGNIFICANT OTHERS

Dispelling myths and offering sexual information should begin with the spinal cord injury patient, but does not always end there. It must often extend to partners and significant others. Partners and family members often have the same misconceptions as the patient. Without proper education they are apt to compound the problem indirectly and unwittingly. Partners often worry about hurting the individual physically or emotionally. They try to avoid being placed in an embarrassing or compromising situation where, once confronted with these limitations, both partners may feel lost. The net result is avoidance.

Some partners are anxious to help with the personal care that the patient needs prior to sexual activity; others may be repelled by the prospect. In either case, these partners are frequently unable to share their reactions for fear of being intrusive or offensive. Thus, they often hesitate in looking for direction and do not take any initiative. The disabled partner often interprets this hesitancy as a sign of rejection, and the lack of clear communication between the parties may lead to a total breakdown in the sexual component of the relationship.

Open and direct channels of communication between partners is a critical component in reaching a sexually satisfying relationship.

FERTILITY IN SPINAL-CORD-INJURED MALES

As noted, fertility is often a major concern for spinal-cord-injured males and is a potential source of anguish. Most research indicates that fertility is low among males with spinal cord injury. Statistical estimates of fertility range between 1% and 10%.[1,3,9,17] As many as 35% of patients report successful efforts at coitus, and 75% to 90% report that they experience reflexogenic or psychogenic erections.[19,26]

Factors accounting for the low incidence of fertility are detailed in the chapter by Mehlman and will not be reviewed here. It is sufficient to state that the incidence of infertility is certainly greatest in complete lesions of the spinal cord and that it diminishes significantly in those patients with incomplete cord lesions. Paraplegic and paraparetic individuals more often experience reflexogenic erections, while a number of quadriparetics often have sacral sparing allowing them at least some partial psychogenic input to sexual arousal.

Many clinicians take a wait-and-see attitude as far as sexual potency in male spinal cord injury patients is concerned. Most of these clinicians also give the individual some understanding of the possible impact of the disability and the statistical probabilities reported in the literature. While many might postulate that a diminution in sexual activity should correlate positively with increasing levels of sexual impairment, the literature indicates that there is no direct correlation between the amount of residual motor function and the level of sexual activity.[15]

SEXUAL CONCERNS OF THE SPINAL-CORD-INJURED FEMALE

Fertility is usually an early concern of the spinal-cord-injured female, but the literature notes that fertility is not impaired. Communication of this information often allays related fears. Basic information on the common post-traumatic reactions, such as the fact that amenorrhea is frequently seen for the first few months after injury, often resolves the patient's concerns.

Once these basic concerns are addressed, the woman with spinal cord injury often confronts other concerns about her sexuality and sexual desirability. Muscle atrophy and other changes often lead to significant concerns about appearance. Many women tend to either reject themselves as sexual beings, or they become much more self-conscious. These women are also concerned about their ability to provide for or serve as an effective mother to their children. These questions often form the crux of their concerns about sexuality once the initial fears have abated.

ORGASM AND EJACULATION

In the spinal-cord-injured male the literature effectively argues that orgasm needs to be distinguished from ejaculation.[10] Ejaculation is often equated with orgasm but does not take into account the added psychological components of the latter. This lack of precision clouds any analysis of how many spinal cord injury patients experience an orgasm that is not associated with ejaculation. There are researchers who believe that orgasm can occur as a pure response of the central nervous system without a peripheral neuromuscular component.[10] This has been confirmed by research on both able-bodied and disabled persons.

Early descriptions of the orgasmic response in the spinal cord injured speak of a "phantom orgasm."[18] This orgasm was described as more cognitively based and was not allied with any genital or pelvic response or sensation. However, the term *phantom* has come under criticism recently. These experiences are deemed to be genuine and are not imagined as the term might imply.

The experience of orgasm devoid of genital or pelvic sensation or response has been reported increasingly by spinal-cord-injured persons. A recent study reported that 30 of 31 individuals surveyed experienced orgasm. Many of these subjects also reported some nondescript subjective genital sensation, although data from neurologic examinations reported no findings of any genital sensation. This may be brought about by the use of some type of cognitive imagery. Individuals reporting such sensation may be drawing upon old recollections of physical sensations that they can now cognitively evoke.

It therefore appears that sexual dysfunction is only one factor mitigating sexual satisfaction and that spinal cord injury patients often can "identify new and gratifying ways of sexual fulfillment."[23(p. 189)]

SECONDARY EROGENOUS ZONES

According to several researchers, many spinal cord injury patients report the development of alternative, highly erogenous and sensitive areas of their bodies after the onset of the disability.[4, 22] Stimulation of these newfound areas seems to heighten sexual arousal, for reasons that are unknown. Such stimulation is therefore often reported to be extremely pleasurable. Many men and women with spinal cord injury report that they experience heightened sensation in their breasts or the area of the mouth and that proper stimulation of such areas leads to a sensation of orgasm. This occurs, possibly, as a result of the concomitant psychological excitation.[25]

Sexual readjustment often requires a willingness to reevaluate what the individual commonly describes as emotionally and sexually exciting along with the willingness to redefine sexual behavior and activity. Ideally, the result of this readjustment is a combination of altered sexual response and the experiencing of new sensations that are stimulating and agreeable.

SEXUAL BEHAVIOR AND SPONTANEITY— PREPARING FOR SEX

Spontaneity is often lost because of the need to take care of several personal grooming activities prior to sexual activity. However, this does not mean that there is an interruption of passion or that there necessarily needs to be a period of sexual inactivity during the time that a spinal-cord-injured individual prepares for sexual contact. This issue needs to be explored with each patient and his partner. In some cases the partner may assist the individual in undressing, bowel and bladder care, positioning, etc., in the process of preparing for sexual activity. In other cases, the use of an attendant for personal care is necessary.

In any case, the process of preparing for sexual activity needs to be discussed openly with both parties, and a trial period needs to be offered as part of ongoing sexual counseling. There are reports in the literature that specifically address self-care activities in preparing for sex, including a well-formulated account of bowel and bladder care.[13]

TIMING SEX EDUCATION AND COUNSELING

When and how should the issues of sexuality be addressed? The best approach seems to be one in which the issues are broached early. However, details should not be pushed upon the patient until he begins to show some concern in this regard. A sensitive, direct statement such as "At some point you may have some questions about sexuality. Please feel free to approach me with such common concerns at any time" may be sufficient at first. If the patient allows a significant period of time to pass after the initial injury—for instance, if hospital discharge is nearing without questions about sexuality—the clinician may need to help by reopening the subject. Where applicable, permission to involve significant others should always be requested and the reasons for this request clearly explained. In a supportive climate, most patients can benefit from specific information and can then apply it fruitfully to enhance their sexual readjustment.

The process of sex education needs to allow for time to digest, experiment, and adjust both behavior and attitudes. It should therefore be done over a period of time that allows for several discussions. The clinician can facilitate the process by sensitively introducing issues and opening areas of blocked discussion as has been described in several theoretical models developed for sexuality counseling.[2, 5, 16]

SEX EDUCATION AND COUNSELING TECHNIQUES

Behavioral rehearsal and role playing can be valuable techniques in helping an individual to express himself socially or to a prospective partner.[27] As the disabled person learns to tactfully educate his audience, he will begin to change his attitudes in a more positive direction and will feel a greater sense of control over his social environment. This can help build the confidence so necessary for effective self-assertiveness.

Learning to be sexually assertive can be very helpful to the individual with a spinal cord injury. Achieving sexual assertiveness can help such a person to feel a sense of mastery over his psychosexual interests, desires, and expressions.[8] Training in sexual assertiveness is usually offered after about six months of disability, once the patient is past his initial reactions toward his disability. At this point he is beginning to deal with issues of separation from the hospital environment and has concerns about returning to the mainstream of society.

CONCLUSION

Adjusting to a spinal cord injury is a difficult and multifaceted process. Sexuality is one of the most important concerns in this process of readjustment. The individual usually begins by focusing on his many physical losses; subsequently the issues of sexuality become more pronounced.

As the spinal cord injury patient goes through the process of preparing for discharge from the hospital and begins to face the monumental task of reentering society, his concerns about social, personal, and sexual life begin to take on more and more significance in contrast to concerns over specific physical disabilities.

Although concern about sexuality may not be a primary focus initially for either the disabled patient or the physician, it is important and should not be totally ignored. Sex education should gradually begin at the early stages following trauma. As discharge approaches, referrals should be made to community agencies such as Planned Parenthood clinics, outpatient urology clinics, and so on.

The patient with a spinal cord injury is frequently overwhelmed with anxieties and fears initially. He often grieves over many losses. Concentration on sexuality may, to the uninitiated, only appear to be adding another burden to the recently injured patient. The point that should be stressed, however, is that no matter how severe the physical limitations, if the patient is willing to explore his body and is willing to overcome his initial fears and frustrations, he may well return to a fulfilling sexual life. Sexuality in the spinal cord injury patient is an issue that needs to be approached openly and that requires a willingness to explore new alternatives and approaches in the quest for satisfaction.

REFERENCES

1. American Association of Sex Educators, Counselors, and Therapists: *Sexual Education, Counseling and Therapy for the Physically Handicapped.* Washington, D.C., 1979.
2. Bedrock G.: *The Care and Management of Spinal Cord Injuries.* New York, Springer-Verlag, 1981.

3. Burke D., Murray D.: *Handbook of Spinal Cord Medicine.* New York, Raven Press, 1975.
4. Cole T.: Spinal cord injury patients and sexual function. *Arch. Phys. Med. Rehabil.* 56:11, 1975.
5. Cole T., Chilgren R., Rosenberg P.: A new program of sex education and counseling for spinal cord injured adults and health care professionals. *Paraplegia* 11:111, 1973.
6. Conine T., Disher C., Gilmore S., et al.: Physical therapists' knowledge of sexuality of adults with spinal cord injury. *Phys. Ther.* 59:395–398, 1979.
7. Dew A., Lynch K., Ernst J., et al.: Reaction and adjustment to spinal cord injury: A descriptive study. *J. Appl. Rehabil. Couns.* 14:32–39, 1983.
8. Dunn M., Lloyd E., Phelps G.: Sexual assertiveness in spinal cord injury. *Sexuality and Disability* 2:293–300, 1979.
9. Eisenberg M., Rustad L.: Sex education and counseling program on a spinal cord injury service. *Arch. Phys. Med. Rehabil.* 57:135–140, 1976.
10. Geiger G.: Neurophysiology of sexual response in spinal cord injury. *Sexuality and Disability* 2:257–266, 1979.
11. Gregory M.: Sexual adjustment: A guide for the spinal cord injured, doctoral dissertation. Bloomington, Il. Accent Special Publications, 1974.
12. Hanson R., Franklin M.: Sexual loss in relation to other functional losses for spinal cord injured males. *Arch. Phys. Med. Rehabil.* 57:291, 1976.
13. Hendrick S.: Spinal cord injury: A special kind of loss. *The Personnel and Guidance Journal* 59:355–359, 1981.
14. Kaplan S.: Sexual counseling for persons with spinal cord injuries: A literature review. *J. Appl. Rehabil. couns.* 10:200–203, 1979.
15. Larsen E., Hejgaard N.: Sexual dysfunction after spinal cord or cauda equina lesions. *Paraplegia* 22:66–74, 1984.
16. Madorsky J., Dixon T.: Rehabilitation aspects of human sexuality. *West. J. Med.* 139:174–176, 1983.
17. Melnyk R., Montgomery R., Over R.: Attitude change following a sexual counseling program for spinal cord injured persons. *Arch. Phys. Med. Rehabil.* 60:601–605, 1979.
18. Money J.: Phantom orgasm in the dreams of paraplegic men and women. *Arch. Gen. Psychiatry* 3:373, 1960.
19. Neiman H.: Venography in acute spinal cord injury, in Calenoff L. (ed.): *Radiology of Spinal Cord Injury.* St. Louis, C.V. Mosby Co., 1981.

20. O'Sullivan S., Cullen K., Smith T.: *Physical Rehabilitation: Evaluation and Treatment Procedures.* Philadelphia, F.A. Davis Co., 1981.
21. Phelps G., Brown M., Chen J., et al.: Sexual experience and plasma testosterone levels in male veterans after spinal cord injury. *Arch. Phys. Med. Rehabil.* 64:47, 1983.
22. Robbins K.: Traumatic spinal cord injury and its impact upon sexuality. *J. Appl. Rehabil. Couns.* 16:24–31, 1985.
23. Sjogren K., Egberg K.: The sexual experience in younger males with complete spinal cord injury. *Scand. J. Rehabil. Med.* 9(suppl.):189–194, 1983.
24. Talbot H.: Psycho-sexual aspects of sexuality in spinal cord injured patients. *Paraplegia* 9:37, 1971.
25. Thornton C.: Sexuality counseling of women with spinal cord injuries. *Sexuality and Disability* 2:267–277, 1979.
26. Verkuyl A.: Sexual function in paraplegia and tetraplegia, in Virken P., Bruyn G. (eds.): *Handbook of Clinical Neurology: Injuries of the Spine and Spinal Cord.* Oxford, North Holland Publishing Co., 1976, vol. 26, pt. 2.
27. Weinberg J.: Human sexuality and spinal cord injury. *Nurs. Clin. North Am.* 17:407–418, 1982.

16

Hospital and Office Management of the Quadriplegic

IN ADDITION TO the diagnosis and treatment of the complicated clinical problems described in the previous chapters, there are many more mundane but nevertheless very important situations that require day-to-day attention both in a hospital and office setting.

As discussed previously, apparently harmless and minor disturbances in nonquadriplegics may assume life-threatening proportions in the quadriplegic patient. Such entities as constipation, upper respiratory tract infection, mild urinary tract infection, and rashes require prophylactic measures in the quadriplegic. However, they also require prompt, efficient therapy so that an apparently minor problem does not ultimately become a life-threatening one.

HOSPITAL MANAGEMENT

With increasingly sophisticated medical care resulting in increased life expectancy in the spinal cord injury patient, it is not uncommon for these patients to have multiple hospital admissions within their life span. Commonly, these readmissions

173

include urologic workup, flap surgery for decubitus ulcer, or therapy for respiratory, vascular, and intestinal complications. Although these problems have been discussed in the chapters devoted to disturbances of specific organ systems in the quadriplegic, it may be worthwhile to spend some additional time on the mechanism of ward management with specific attention to order writing, supervision of house staff, and supervision of nursing and ancillary personnel. Some attention must also be paid to indications for the obtaining of consultation. It is also necessary to examine the relationship of the spinal cord injury patient and those responsible for his care to the hospital at large.

BASIC MAINTENANCE CARE

Even in the "nonsick" quadriplegic (in other words, a patient who has no acute current medical problems) certain basic issues must be addressed on a day-to-day basis. These include the following:

Skin Care

Spinal cord injury patients require side-to-side bed positioning with frequent turning, preferably every two hours. Positioning in bed should avoid excess flexion of the extremities, and in some cases upper and/or lower extremity positioning splints may be required. Lower extremity resting splints are preferable to so-called bed boards, which encourage poor positioning of the feet.

The surface of the bed should be made as soft as possible with a firm underlying base. Examples of such mattresses are egg crate mattresses, full sheepskin covers, or water/gel beds. More cumbersome electric or specialized beds are not required in every case. This is fortunate in that basic hospital beds can easily be converted for use in the quadriplegic patient.

Daily skin checks should be done either by physicians or by nursing staff. Signs of erythema or minor abrasions demand immediate attention as an indication for change of position to avoid any pressure to the area. In most cases decubiti can be prevented by scrupulous and frequent inspection of the skin. Decubitus care has been covered in detail in the chapter on dermatology.

Bladder

The method of urinary drainage and the scheduling of intermittent catheterization should be clearly outlined in admission orders. Many patients may also require medication for the maintenance of integrity of the urinary tract such as antimicrobial and antispasmodic drugs.

Adequate drainage of the urinary tract is of course essential in preventing crisis caused by urinary retention. Medical and nursing staff should be alerted to the presenting signs of autonomic dysreflexia, which notably include high blood pressure, bradycardia, and sweating.

Bowel

The patient's individual bowel routine should be continued while in the hospital; otherwise, one runs the risk of impaction with attendant autonomic crisis. Initiation of a bowel routine in the new quadriplegic has proven to be equally efficacious in the prevention of crisis.

Respiratory Tract

When a spinal cord injury patient is admitted, even if he has no acute respiratory problems, the staff should be made aware of the need for assistive cough. Attention should also be directed to the arising of acute respiratory problems during admission for nonrespiratory reasons—an occurrence that is not infrequent. Alertness to the problem and prompt management will frequently obviate prolonged, debilitating, and often serious respiratory infections.

Vascular

In view of the frequent appearance of deep venous thrombosis with or without pulmonary embolism in the immobilized quadriplegic, a significant degree of alertness to the appearance of one or both of the above should be exercised by physicians and nursing staff alike. However, since deep venous thrombosis can be very occult, the use of prophylactic subcutaneous heparin (miniheparin) should be considered on admission of quadriplegics for other than active vascular problems. Obviously, full-scale heparinization must be utilized for cases of deep venous thrombosis.

Table 16–1 demonstrates a typical set of basic admission orders for a quadriplegic patient. These orders obviously do not include provisions for care of specific problems that have been adequately covered in the chapters on disorders of specific organ systems in the quadriplegic.

OFFICE MANAGEMENT

Nothing is better testimony to the increased sophistication of medical care of the quadriplegic than the longevity and quality of life in these patients in current times. There would have been no need 40 years ago for a section on office management of the quadriplegic, since these patients either died soon after the precipitating event or spent the rest of their lives in a closely supervised fashion. Currently, quadriplegics may live at home, go to school, and may well drive themselves to the doctor's office in customized vehicles. It is hoped that with even further refinement of care it will be possible in the future to provide most of the medical care of the quadriplegic in a doctor's office with only a rare hospitalization for unusual illness.

Barring acute illnesses that require immediate evaluation (a quadriplegic with a complaint should be seen on the same day) it is adequate for the usual quadriplegic to be routinely examined twice a year. At this time a general physical examination should be performed as on any other patient. Histori-

TABLE 16–1.—Basic Admission orders for the Quadriplegic Patient

Diagnosis—Quadriplegia
Condition—Good
Activity—(1) Turning side to side q2h
          (2) Egg crate mattress
          (3) Transfer o.o.b to chair with assistance
          (4) Upper-extremity splints placed h.s.
Diet—regular
Allergy—– – – – – –
Vitals—q. shift
Condom catheter drainage—Intermittent catheterization t.i.d.
Bowel routine—Performed h.s. with suppositories
Medications—(1) Miniheparin, 5,000 units sc q12hr
             (2) Colace, 100 mg. p.o. t.i.d.
             (3) Senokot, ii p.o. b.i.d.
             (4) Therevac suppository rectally qhs
             (5) Probanthine, 15 mg. p.o. t.i.d.
             (6) Baclofen, 20 mg. p.o. b.i.d.
             (7) Mandelamine, i gm p.o. q.i.d.
             (8) Vitamin C, 500 mg p.o. q.i.d.
Chest x-ray
Bloods—SMA6, CBC P.T., P.T.T., ESR, total protein albumin
ECG
Urinalysis
Call M.D. if increased blood pressure or diminished heart rate or sweating
Assistive cough if dysphagia or choking occurs
Daily skin check
Physical therapy as ordered
Active assistive range of motion/passive range of motion all four extremities daily

cally, specific attention should be paid to (1) residual volumes and intermittent catheterization or change in the appearance of the urine; (2) success of the bowel regimen; (3) degree of spasticity; (4) frequency of autonomic crisis; and (5) frequency of upper respiratory tract infection.

Special attention on physical examination should be paid to (1) integrity of the skin; (2) degree of spasticity; (3) development of any new contractures; (4) evidence of fecal impaction; and (5) change in respiratory status.

Although it is proper to be concerned about any symptoms of which the quadriplegic complains, these patients may also really have minor illnesses, like nonquadriplegic patients. These include the common cold, intercurrent gastroenteritis, and minor trauma such as cuts and bruises. As the physician becomes more and more experienced (and thus more relaxed in the care of these patients) he or she is usually able to separate intercurrent illness without sequelae from intercurrent illness with serious potential at the time of the examination.

Because of the disordered physiology of the spinal cord injury patient, even though one may be facing an active problem involving one system, constant monitoring and evaluation of all other systems is necessary at all times.

Index

Amoxicillin, 81
Amphotericin B, 82
Ampicillin, 81
Amylase, pancreatitis and, 37, 102
Amyloid disease, 132–133
Anal sphincter, 62
Anemia, 158–159
Anesthesia
  epidural, 139
  general, 140–141
  spinal, 139
Anger, 16
Angiography, 121
Ankylosis, 110–111
Anorexia, 104
Antibiotic
  catheterization and, 64
    irrigation and, 76
  gram-negative bacilli and, 56
  intermittent catheterization and, 78–79
  pneumonia and, 52–53
    aspiration, 53–54
    staphylococcal, 56
Anticholinergic drug, 139
Anticoagulation, 121–123
  bleeding and, 123–124
  pulmonary embolus and, 124
Anuria, 84
Anxiety, 18
Apnea, sleep, 39
Appendicitis, 103
Architectural accessibility, 20
ARDS; see Acute respiratory distress syndrome
Areflexic bladder, 62, 63
Arterial blood gases, 58–59

Artery syndrome, superior mesenteric, 102–103
Aspiration
  diagnosis of, 51–52
  gastric contents and, 38
  pneumonia and, 53–55
Aspirin, 122
Assertiveness, self, 169
Assisted cough, 40
Asymptomatic bacteriuria, 74
  treatment of, 77–78
Atelectasis
  incentive spirometry and, 40–41
  lobar, 34
  secretion retention and, 36
  segmental, 34
Atrophy, muscle, 118
Atropine, 33
Autistic-like reaction, 18
Autonomic crisis, 137–140
  gastrointestinal tract and, 98
Autonomic dysreflexia, 71
  labor and, 90
Autonomic hyperreflexia, 69–70
  fecal impaction and, 104

B

Bacilli, gram-negative, 56–58
Baclofen, 115
Bacteremia, 55
Bacterial pneumonia
  aspiration, 54
  suppurative, 52
Bacteriuria
  asymptomatic, 74

Burst fracture, 7–8
Button, tracheostomy, 44

C

Cachexia, 118
Calculi
  renal, 84
    catheterization and, 74
    intermittent
      catheterization and, 75
  urinary, 157–158
Calorie, 157
Candida
  antibiotic treatment and,
    82
  cystitis and, 79
Capacitance, venous, 139
Carbenicillin, 83
Cardiac arrest, 140
Cardiac reflex, 139
Cardiac tamponade, 37
Cardiopulmonary
    complications, 25–50;
    see also Circulatory
    complications;
    Respiratory tract
Cast, white blood cell, 80
Catecholamines, 36
Catheter; *see also*
    Catheterization
  condom, 68
  curved-tip, 35
  Foley, 74–76, 82
  care of, 75–77
  infection and, 73–74
  indwelling, 63
  obstructed, 76
  straight suction, 35

suprapubic, 65
Swan-Ganz, 33, 37,
  140–141
Catheterization, intermittent;
  see also Catheter
  follow-up and, 65
  infection and, 78–79
  spinal shock and, 63
Caustic solution, 132
Cefadroxil, 81
Cefazolin, 55
Cefoperazone, 57
Ceftazidime, 57
Central cervical spinal cord
  syndrome, 3
Central respiratory centers,
  28
Cephalexin
  pyogenic bacterial
    pneumonia and, 55
  urinary tract infection and,
    81
Cephalosporin
  pneumonia and, 57
  urinary tract infection and,
    81, 82
Cephalothin, 55, 56
Cephapirin, 55, 56
Cephradine, 81
Cervical spinal cord
  syndrome, 3
Cervical spine
  bony injury and, 6–8
  upper, 1–2
Cervical traction, 6
Chemical pneumonitis,
  53–54
Chest
  percussion, 40
  physical therapy and,
    39–41

trauma and, 37
vibration and, 40
x-ray and, 58–59
Chest cavity, 30–31
Chest wall mechanics, 28
Circulatory complications,
137–146
autonomic crisis and,
137–140
general anesthesia and,
140–141
postural hypertension and,
141–143
Clavicle, 3
Clindamycin
pneumonia and, 54
pyogenic bacterial
pneumonia and, 55
Clotting system, 117–118
Cocci, gram-positive, 54
Colonization vs.
superinfection, 58–59
Complication
of aspiration pneumonia,
54–55
circulatory, 137–146
endocrine, 147–153
gastrointestinal, 95–108
ileus as, 98
musculoskeletal, 109–116
skin and, 127–133
respiratory, 25–50
thrombosis and, 117–126
urinary tract infections
and, 83–84
Compression, evaluation of, 5
Compression fracture, 7
Computed tomography, 4
neurologic deficit and, 5
osteomyelitis and, 129
osteoporosis and, 112

Conditioning, operant, 42
Condom catheter, 68
Cone
of edema, 39
of hemorrhage, 39
Consciousness, 30
Constipation, 139
Contraction
bladder, 67
diaphragmatic, 25–26
muscle, 113–114
Coordinated sphincter
management of, 67–68
postrecovery phase and, 66
Cost of spinal cord injury, 12
Cough, 29–30
assisted, 40
Coumadin
deep vein thrombosis and,
122
pulmonary embolus and,
124–125
Counseling, sex, 162,
168–169
Crisis, hypertensive
autonomic, 139
intraoperative, 141
Crutchfield tongs, 6
CT scan; see Computed
tomography
Cuirass, 45
Culture
pneumonia and, 54
sputum, 52, 58
urine, 64
catheterization and, 77
follow-up and, 65
hyperreflexic bladder, 68
urinary tract infection
and, 80
Curved-tip catheter, 35

Cutaneous vesicostomy, 65
Cystitis
    antibiotics and, 80–83
    Candida and, 79
    enterococcal, 81
Cystometry, 66
Cystostomy, 63, 65

D

Dantrolene sodium, 114
Debridement, 132
Decompression, gastric or
    intestinal, 32
Decubitus ulcer, 127–133
    autonomic crisis and, 139
    heterotopic ossification
        and, 111
Deep venous thrombosis,
    110, 117–121
    hospital management and,
        176
    treatment of, 121–125
Deformity, spinal, 113
Denial, 16, 17–18, 20–21
Depression, 17, 18, 19
Dermatitis, 133
Desire, sexual, 163
Detrusor-sphincter
    dyssynergia, 71
Detrusor muscle, 63
Diabetes, 77–78
Diagnostic peritoneal lavage,
    98
Diaphragm
    contraction and, 25–26
    innervation and, 2
    pacing of, 45–46
    paralysis and, 39

phrenic nerve stimulation
    and, 45–46
Diarrhea, 104
Diazepam, 114
Diet, 155–160
    low-calcium, 157
Dilatation, gastric,
Diplococci
    pneumonia and, 55
    sputum and, 52
Dislocation, facet, 7
Disodium editronate
    diphosphonate,
        111–112
Distention, abdominal, 97–98
Distress, acute respiratory,
    36–37
    intubation and, 32
Ditropan
    autonomic crisis and, 139
    hyperreflexic bladder with
        coordinated sphincter
        and, 68
Diuretic
    acute respiratory distress
        syndrome and, 37
    extremity edema and, 156
Diverticulum, 75
Dopamine beta-hydroxylase,
    142
Doppler test, 120
Doppler ultrasound flow
    detector, 119
Drainage
    bladder, 65
    postural, 40
    tidal, 65
Duodenum
    superior mesenteric artery
        syndrome and, 102
    ulcer and, 101

Dysfunction, voiding, 61–72
Dysreflexia, 69
  autonomic, 71
  labor and, 90
Dyssynergia
  detrusor-sphincter, 71
  internal sphincter, 66,
    68–70
  vesico-urethral, 68

E

Early evaluation, 30–31
ECV; *see* Extracellular volume
Edema
  cone of, 39
  leg, 118
    extracellular volume
      and, 156
    noncardiogenic pulmonary,
      36–37
  pulmonary, 31, 37
    anesthesia and, 140
Effusion, pleural, 52
Ejaculation, 89, 166–167
Electromyography of external
    sphincter, 66
Embolus
  pulmonary, 117, 118
    diagnosis of, 120
    hospital management
      and, 176
    treatment of, 124–125
  fat, 38
Emotional factors, 11–24
Emphysema, 30
Empyema, 55
Endocrine complication,
    147–153

glucose metabolism and,
    151
gonadal abnormality and,
    151–152
hypercalcemia and,
    147–150
thyroid dysfunction and,
    150–151
Endotracheal intubation,
    32–33
  bradycardia and, 140
  cardiac arrest and, 140
  tracheostomy and, 44
Enteric bacilli, 56–57
Enterobacter, 56
Enterococcus
  antibiotic treatment and,
    82
  cystitis and, 81
  urinary tract infection and,
    79
Environment
  barrier removal and, 20
  emotional shock and, 15
Epidemiology, 12–14
Epidural anesthesia, 139
Equal access, 20
Erection, 88–89
Erogenous zone, 167–168
Erosion
  gastric, 101
  penile prosthetic device
    and, 93
ERV; *see* Expiratory reserve
    volume
Erythromycin, 55
Erythropoietin, 158–159
Escherichia coli, 56
  urinary tract infection and,
    79
Ethacrynic acid, 149

radiographic evaluation and, 4
rib, 31
vertebral body, 7–8
FRC; *see* Functional residual capacity
Frog breathing, 42
Functional residual capacity, 27
Fungal infection, 134
Furosemide, 149
Fusobacterium nucleatum, 54

G

Ganglionic blocking agent, 141
autonomic crisis and, 139
Gardner-Wells tongs, 6
Gas exchange, 27–28
Gastric contents, aspiration of, 38
Gastric dilatation, 53
Gastric erosion, 101
Gastrin, 99
Gastrointestinal complications, 95–108
appendicitis and, 103
clinical aspects of, 96–97
fecal impaction and, 104–105
gastroparesis and, 99
hemorrhage and, 100–101
anticoagulation therapy and, 123
ventilator and, 34
ileus and, 98–99
innervation of bowel, 95–96

pancreatitis and, 102
symptoms and findings of, 97–98
stress ulcer and, 99–100
superior mesenteric artery syndrome and, 102–103
Gastroparesis, 99
General anesthesia, 140–141
Gentamicin, 82
Globulin, 150
Glossopharyngeal breathing, 42
Glucose, 151
Gonadal abnormality, 151–152
Gonadotrophin, 152
Gram-negative organism bacilli, 56–58
rod, 54
urinary tract infection and, 83
Gram-positive organism cocci, 54, 55–56
urinary tract infection and, 79, 83
Gram's stain
pneumonia and, 54
sputum, 52
urine and, 79–80
Guanethidine, 139
Gulp, 42
Gynecomastia, 152

H

Halo ring, 6
Halothane, 141
Halo-vest immobilization facet dislocation and, 7

I

Intubation *(cont.)*
    cardiac arrest and, 140
    tracheostomy and, 44, 45
    nasogastric, 44
Inversine, 139
Iodine-121 scan, 119
IPPB; *see* Intermittent positive pressure breathing
Irrigation, 35
Ischemia, 128
Ischial tuberosity, 130

K

Kidney; *see also* Urinary tract
    calculi and, 74, 75, 84
    damage and, 84
Klebsiella
    pneumonia and, 56
    urinary tract infection and, 79
Kubler-Ross, 16–18
Kyphosis, 113
    decubitus ulcer and, 130
    osteoporosis and, 112

L

Labor, 90
Lavage, 35
    diagnostic peritoneal, 98
Left heart failure, 36–37
Leg edema, 118
Lesion, 131–132
Libido, 163
    male and, 88

Lidocaine, 115
Lipase, 38
Lobar atelectasis, 34
Long-term care, 43–44
    ventilatory assistance and, 44–45
Lordosis, 113
Low-calcium diet, 157
Lung abscess, 55
Lung volumes, 27

M

Male
    fertility and, 165–166
    immobilization hypercalcemia and, 148, 158
    risk factor and, 12–13
    sexual potential and, 87–89
Malnutrition, 155
Management, hospital, of spinal injured, 173–176
Maximal midexpiratory flow, 28
Maximum breathing capacity, 28
MBC; *see* Maximum breathing capacity
Mechanical ventilation, 33–34
Mechanics, respiratory, 28–29
Mecomylamine, 139
Menstruation, 152
Mesenteric artery syndrome, superior, 102–103

Metabolism, glucose, 151
Methicillin, 56
Microembolus, 38
Microglobule, fat, 38
Micturition
  fluoroscopic study of, 66
  hyperreflexic bladder with
    dyssynergic sphincter
    and, 68
Mini-heparin therapy,
  121–123
Minipress, 70
Motor vehicle injury, 13
Mucoid impaction, 34–35
Mucolytic, 35
Mucomyst, 34–35
Muscle; see also
  Musculoskeletal
  complications
  atrophy and, 118
  detrusor, 63
  intercostal, 26
  lesions penetrating to,
    132–133
  respiratory, 25–27
    paralysis and, 2
    rehabilitation of, 42
  spasticity and, 113–114
Musculoskeletal
  complications,
  109–116
  heterotopic ossification
    and, 109–112
  muscle and, 113–116
  osteomyelitis and,
    112–113
  osteoporosis and, 112
  skeletal deformity and,
    113
Myelogram, 5
Myositis ossificans, 109

N

$Na_2H_3PO_4$, 149
Nafcillin, 56
Nalidixic acid, 81
Nasogastric tube, 31–32
Nasotracheal tube, 44
Neck
  bladder, 70
  examination of, 30
  innervation and, 3
Necrosis
  acute tubular, 84
  ischial tuberosity and, 130
  pressure-related, 128
Necrotizing pneumonia,
  54–55
Nerve
  pudendal, 96
  root and, 2
  vagus, 95–96
Nerve block
  hyperreflexic bladder with
    coordinated sphincter
    and, 68
  spasticity and, 115–116
Neurogenic bladder, 61–72
  acute phase and, 62
  follow-up and, 65
  hyperreflexic bladder and,
    67–70
  management of, 63–65, 67
  pharmacologic
    management and, 70
  postrecovery phase and, 66
  unbalanced function and,
    70–71
  urodynamic findings and,
    62
Neurogenic bowel, 95

Neurologic deficit,
incomplete, 8
radiographic evaluation
and, 5
Neurologic examination, 1
Nitrofurantoin, 81
Noncardiogenic pulmonary
edema, 36–37
Nontouch technique of
catheterization, 75
Nutrition, 155–160

O

Obstruction
catheter, 76
duodenal, 102
Occult bleeding, 123
Oliguria, 64
Open wound in chest wall,
31
Operant conditioning, 42
Oral anticoagulants, 123
Orders, admission, 177
Orgasm, 89, 166–167
female, 89
phantom, 167
Orotracheal tube, 44
Orthostatic hypotension, 141
Ossification, 109–112
Osteomyelitis, 112–113
decubitus ulcer and, 129
deep lesion and, 132
Osteoporosis, 112
Overdistention of bladder, 63
Overload, circulatory,
140–141
acute, 37
Oxacillin, 56
Oxybutynin, 68

P

Pacing of diaphragm, 45–46
Packing, decubitus ulcer and,
132
$PaCO_2$, 33
Pain
gastrointestinal, 96–97
shoulder
pancreatitis and, 102
perforation of
gastrointestinal tract
and, 100
Palm, 3
Palpation, rectal, 104
Pancreatitis, 37, 102
PaO_2, 33
Paradoxical rib cage motion,
28
Paralysis
diaphragmatic, 39
total respiratory muscle, 2
Paralytic ileus, 98
Parasympathetic stimulus,
140
Parathyroid hormone, 148
Parenteral hyperalimentation,
156
Partner, sexual, 164–165
PCO_2, 28
Peak flow, 28
PEEP; *see* Positive and
expiratory pressure
Penetrating wound, 13
Penicillin
penicillinase-resistant, 56
pneumonia and, 54, 55
Penile prosthetic device, 91,
93
Pentolinium, 141
autonomic crisis and, 139

Psychological adjustment
(cont.)
epidemiology of injury and,
12–14
initial, 14–15
sexuality and, 161–172; see
also Sexual function
theories of, 15–20
Pudendal nerve, 96
Pulmonary angiography, 121
Pulmonary complication, 98;
see also Respiratory
tract
Pulmonary edema, 31, 37
anesthesia and, 140
hypoxemia and, 36
noncardiogenic, 36–37
Pulmonary embolism, 117,
118
diagnosis of, 120
hospital management and,
176
treatment of, 124–125
Pulmonary toilet, 29–30
pneumonia and, 53
Purulent sputum, 52
Pyelonephritis, 83, 84
Pyogenic bacterial
pneumonia, 55–59

R

Race as risk factor, 13
Radiograph
acute respiratory
deterioration and, 34
evaluation and, 4–5, 31
respiratory compromise
and, 36–37

ulcer perforation and, 100
Rales, 31
Range of motion
deep vein thrombosis and,
122
heterotopic ossification
and, 110–111
Rectal palpation, 104
Reduction of facet
dislocation, 7
Referred pain, 97
Reflex, 139; see also
Hyperreflexia;
Hyperreflexic bladder
Reflux
ureteral, 75
urine, 69
Rehabilitation
centers for, 92
inspiratory resistive
breathing and, 42–43
sexual, 90–91
Renal calculi, 84
catheterization and, 74
intermittent catheterization
and, 75
Renal damage, 84
Renal shutdown, 83–84
Residual volume
bladder
autonomic crisis and,
139
post-void, 67–68
unbalanced function and,
70–71
lung, 27
Resin, hydrophyllic, 132
Respiratory tract, 25–50
acute care and, 30–39
evaluation and, 30–31
initial care and, 31–32

Serum amylase, 37, 102
Serum dopamine beta-
    hydroxylase, 142
Serum T₄ level, 150
Serum total protein, 131
Sex as risk factor, 13
Sexual function
    desire and, 163
    education and counseling
        and, 168–169
    fears about, 163–164
    female and, 89–90, 166
    fertility and, 165–166
    male and, 87–89
        options for, 91, 93
    orgasm and ejaculation
        and, 166–167
    partner and, 164–165
    rehabilitation and, 90–91
    secondary erogenous zones
        and, 167–168
    spontaneity and, 168
Shock
    emotional, 14–15
    spinal, 3
        fluid resuscitation in, 37
        reaction and, 20
Shoulder pain
    pancreatitis and, 102
    perforation of
        gastrointestinal tract
        and, 100
Sigh, 29
Significant other, 164–165
Silicone catheter, 76–77
Silicone implant, penile, 91,
    93
Skeletal complications; see
    Musculoskeletal
    complications
Skin, 127–134
    acne and, 133

alopecia areata and,
    133–134
decubitus ulcer and,
    127–133
fungal infection and, 134
maintenance care and,
    174–175
seborrheic dermatitis and,
    133
Sleep apnea, 39
Sleeping surface, 130
Soak, 122
Social adjustment, 20; see
    also Psychological
    adjustment
Sodium chloride, 149
Sodium restriction, 156
Soft tissue inflammation,
    110
Spasm, 3, 112–114
    abdominal, 97
    cough and, 35
    dyspnea and, 29
    sexual function and, 90
Spermatogenesis, 151–152
Sphincter
    hyperreflexic bladder, 66,
        67–70
    internal urethral, 70
    urinary or anal, 62
Sphincterotomy, 70, 71
Spinal anesthesia, 139
Spinal shock, 3
    bladder and, 62
    fluid resuscitation in, 37
Spine
    deformity of, 113
    initial evaluation of, 1–8
Spirometry, incentive,
    40–41
Splanchnic return, 142
Spontaneous erection, 88

Sports injury, 13
Sputum
    Pneumococcus and, 55
    pneumonia and, 54
    purulent, 52
    superinfection and, 58–59
Stain, Gram's, of sputum, 52
Staphylococcus
    antibiotic treatment and,
        82
    pneumonia and, 54, 55–56
    urinary tract infection and,
        79
Stenosis, subglottic, 44
Sterile intermittent
        catheterization, 63–64
Sterilization, 90
Steroid
    aspiration pneumonia and,
        54
    hypercalcemia and, 148
Stimulation, afferent,
        137–140
Stimulus, 140
Stoma, tracheostomy, 44
Stone
    renal, 84
        catheterization and, 74,
            75
    urinary tract, 157–158
Straight suction catheter, 35
Streptococcus viridans, 54
Stress ulcer, 99–100
Subcutaneous emphysema,
        30
Subcutaneous fat, 128
Subglottic stenosis, 44
Subluxation
    facet dislocation and, 7
    radiographic evaluation
        and, 4
Succinylcholine, 141

Suction catheter, 35
Suctioning
    bradycardia and, 33
    respiratory care and, 31
    tracheal, 35
Sugar, fasting blood, 151
Sulfa, 80
Sulfa-trimethoprim, 81
Sulfisoxazole, 80–81
Superficial excoriation,
        131
Superinfection, 58–59
Superior mesenteric artery
        syndrome, 102–103
Superoxygenation, 33
Suppurative bacterial
        pneumonia, 52
Suprapubic catheter, 65
Suprapubic cystostomy, 65
Surgery, deep lesions and,
        132
Swan-Ganz catheter, 33, 37,
        140–141
Sweat
    autonomic crisis and,
        138
    autonomic hyperreflexia
        and, 69
Swelling; *see* Edema
Sympathetic catecholamines,
        36
Sympathetic reflex
    autonomic crisis and,
        137–140
    injury to, 3
Syndrome
    acute respiratory distress,
        36–37
    central cervical spinal
        cord, 3
    superior mesenteric artery,
        102–103

T

T$_4$ level, 150
Tachycardia, 142
Tamponade, cardiac, 37
Technetium-labeled human
    albumin, 119
Telogen effluvium, 134
Testosterone, 88, 151
Tetracycline, 81
Thermodilution, 141
Thromboembolism,
    121–125
Thromboplastin, 117
    fat, 38
Thrombosis, deep venous,
    110, 117–120
    hospital management and,
    176
    treatment of, 121–125
Thyroid binding globulin,
    150
Thyroid dysfunction,
    150–151
Ticarcillin
    pneumonia and, 57
    pyelonephritis and, 83
Tidal drainage, 65
Tilt table, 142
TLC; *see* Total lung capacity
Tobramycin
    pneumonia and, 57
    urinary tract infection and,
    82
Tomography, computed
    osteomyelitis and, 129
    osteoporosis and, 112
Tongs, 6
Total lung capacity, 27
Total protein, serum, 131

Total respiratory muscle
    paralysis, 2
Tracheal suctioning
    bradycardia and, 140
    cardiac arrest and, 140
    intubation and, 35
Tracheobronchial tree
    pneumonia and, 58
    secretion and, 34
Tracheostomy, 43–44
    long-term, 45
Traction
    cervical, 6
    facet dislocation and, 7
Trauma
    blood transfusion and, 38
    chest, 37
    to nose or mouth, 30
Trigger of voiding, 67
Trimethopan, 139, 141
Tube
    cystostomy, 63
    nasotracheal, 44
    orotracheal, 44
    tracheostomy, 44
Tuberosity, 130
Tubular necrosis, 84
Tunica albuginea, 93
Turning, 129–130

U

Ulcer
    decubitus, 127–133
    stress, 99–100
Upper cervical spine, 1–2
Upper urinary tract infection,
    83
Ureteral reflux, 75

White blood cell *(cont.)*
  superinfection and, 58–59
White matter, 3
Wound
  chest wall, 31
  penetrating, 13

X

X-ray; *see* Radiographic
      evaluation